Ketogenic
Diet
3 BOOKS IN 1
The Complete Healthy And Delicious Recipes Cookbook Box Set
By:*Emily Simmons*

Book one
Ketogenic Diet for Beginners
That You Can Prep In 15 Minutes Or Less
Emily Simmons

KETOGENIC DIET 3 BOOKS IN 1 THE COMPLETE HEALTHY AND DELICIOUS RECIPES COOKBOOK BOX SET 3

Copyright © by Emily Simmons
All rights reserved. No part of this book
May be used or reproduced in any matter
Whatsoever without permission in writing from
The author except in the case of brief quotations
Embodied in critical articles or review.

Disclaimer:

The information presented in this book represents the views of the publisher as of the date of publication. The publisher reserves the rights to alter update their opinions based on new conditions. This report is for informational purposes only. The author and the publisher do not accept any responsibilities for any liabilities resulting from the use of this information. While every attempt has been made to verify the information provided here, the author and the publisher cannot assume any responsibility for errors, inaccuracies or omissions. Any similarities with people or facts are unintentional.

Introduction

A completely new lifestyle is waiting for you! This book is written strictly according to the ketogenic diet. You will find an entire range of ketogenic recipes. If you are new to the ketogenic concept, the basic thing is that this diet plan is based on a high fat and low carbohydrate intake. Thus, do not get intimidated by the cheese and meat recipes in this book if you are presently on a low-fat weight loss regime. Don't worry. We won't tell you anything which makes you gain weight.

We have not kept any secrets about the ketogenic diet. Since it is an entirely new diet, your body will need time to adapt. You'll have to be patient for about 2-3 weeks until it becomes a habit to eat negligible amounts of carbohydrates. But ultimately, you will start feeling good about your body. The energy you get from these foods is mobilized from the fats you receive. You will feel energetic as well as satiated for hours at your workplace or home. Thus, you will not get those cravings for eating so frequently that you get when you are on a high carbohydrate diet.

Carbohydrates do provide energy to your body, but they do not keep you full for long. The fats that are received along with carbohydrates are stored around your stomach and thighs until needed. However, with the ketogenic diet, you do not have to worry while indulging in fatty foods. We will explain to you how the diet works in more detail in section 1 of this book. Therefore, you will not be blindly following the high fat and low carbohydrate diet, but will have a good understanding of how it works.

What is the Ketogenic Diet?

The ketogenic diet is high in fats and moderate in proteins but low in carbohydrates. The diet is typically designed so that the body burns the fat in the food and not the carbohydrates. Hence, the carbohydrate is converted into forms of glucose. The glucose gets transported throughout the body and plays a very important role in the functioning of the brain. This metabolism is called ketosis.

Ketosis is a process that naturally benefits the body. The human body adapts itself to ketosis when food is not available. The same process is utilized in the modern world to lose weight naturally. Ketone bodies show improvement in diseases and thus we naturally stay immune. The diet is used to treat even extreme medical conditions like epilepsy, diabetes, Alzheimer's, autism, cancer, etc.

However, it is highly advised that you do not blindly follow the ketogenic diet plan. There are many different ketogenic diet charts, but you can choose the one which is most suitable for you. The most famous ketogenic diet is the Atkins diet. The main concern of the ketogenic diet is the amount of carbohydrates to be consumed per day. The diet plan is based on the monitoring of the intake of carbohydrates in a day, which is ideally just 20-60 grams. The protein intake is moderate and depends upon how much exercise you do and what your gender and height are. The balance of calories is obtained from fats. Once you start the ketogenic diet, your objective should be to follow it for as long as possible.

The intake of nutrients in a ketogenic plan is as follows: 70-75% of the calories are obtained from fats, 20-25% from proteins and 5-10% from carbohydrates. The calories are unrestricted in such a diet. Your hunger reduces in this diet plan. Thus, it's up to you whether you count your calories or not.

Things to remember before following the ketogenic diet and why should you consume high fat with moderate levels of proteins?

KETOGENIC DIET 3 BOOKS IN 1 THE COMPLETE HEALTHY AND DELICIOUS RECIPES COOKBOOK BOX SET

Fats do not affect blood insulin and sugar levels. Proteins do affect insulin as well as blood sugar if consumed in large quantities. High levels of insulin can restrict the ability of the body to burn and release fatty acids that provide necessary elements required for ketosis. Some people might be affected by it more than others depending upon how much they exercise. Moreover, following a diet with high levels of lean protein and not enough fats might make you ill with a strange health condition called "rabbit starvation". The concept to remember therefore for those who want to lose fat while maintaining blood sugar levels is that you should eat fat to lose more fat.

Targeted Ketogenic Diet and Cyclical Ketogenic Diet

There are two types of diets for people who exercise regularly. The targeted ketogenic diet is one where you consume carbohydrates just before and just after your regime of workouts. This plan suits those who are involved in doing intense workouts daily and require some carbohydrate as fuel.

The cyclical ketogenic diet is one where you consume a minimum amount of carbohydrates per day. On weekends, you consume relatively higher quantities of carbohydrates in order to refill your store of muscle glycogen. This is done to maintain the energy levels in your body for the workouts you do.

Who should follow the ketogenic diet?

Doctors typically recommend this diet for those children whose seizures do not respond to various seizure medicines. Children suffering with Lennox-Gastaut syndrome are particularly prescribed with this medicine.

Usually, adults have not in the past followed these diets. Still, there are many examples, where adults have also benefitted from this. Since there are many live examples around us, the trend of the ketogenic diet is catching on.

Epilepsy conditions in particular may be improved with the ketogenic diet. In brief, anyone can follow this diet unless there are some particular reasons not to follow it.

Benefits of the ketogenic diet

Low carbohydrate diets have been controversial since the time they emerged. However, the fact is that many human studies have proved that they are beneficial in many ways. Let's take a look at some of the benefits:

The ketogenic diet kills excessive appetite for all the right reasons. It makes you feel full for longer.

You can lose weight faster than those on active diet plans.

This diet is very effective in reducing the abdominal fat that is harmful for the body.

It reduces the risk of heart diseases.

Your levels of insulin and blood sugar are improved.

Those suffering with high blood pressure experience improvement.

Many brain disorders are proven to have been cured by ketogenic diets.

Dangers of the ketogenic diet

If you have kidney problems, the high protein levels of the ketogenic diet may worsen the problem.
Kidney stones are likely to get worse due to the excessive urinating of calcium.
If you do not consume fiber in your diet, too much meat may not prove good for your gut health; increased acid formation due to excessive consumption of meat and no fiber.
Again, low consumption of fruits and vegetables causes inflammation.

Side effects of the ketogenic diet
It is a little difficult to switch to the ketogenic diet plan. Therefore it will help to know about a few side effects that you might face in the first week of beginning a ketogenic diet. You can then be prepared for them beforehand and take some precautions to avoid them. It becomes easy to cure the side effects if you know the reasons behind them. Your body needs some time to switch from your regular diet and adjust itself to burn fat and not glucose. It need some time to create some enzymes.

Frequent urination
You might use the bathroom more often than before a day after you start this diet. This is because your body burns glucose that is stored in your muscles and liver. This process releases more water.

Dizziness and fatigue
When your body dumps water, minerals like potassium, salt and magnesium are also lost. This may cause dizziness and fatigue. You can avoid these side effects by consuming more minerals found in various food sources. Drink salty broth or flavor your food with more salt.

Consume foods with more potassium. Leafy vegetables are a major source of potassium.

Make a note to consult your doctor if you are under medication for high blood pressure, kidney ailments or heart diseases.

Low blood sugar

When you have a diet rich in carbohydrates, your body keeps some insulin aside to absorb the sugar which is created from the carbohydrate. But, during the ketogenic diet, you might experience low blood sugar because of lower carbohydrate levels. Eating frequently helps to cure this side effect.

Headache

Due to the loss of a few minerals, you might experience headaches in the initial days. Again, drinking salty broth helps in this condition. If nothing else helps, you may add a little carbohydrate to your diet.

Constipation

Apart from other things, constipation is the most common side effect that happens to the new followers of the ketogenic diet due to an imbalance of magnesium and potassium. You can cut down on your consumption of nuts and drink a lot of water to avoid constipation.

Sugar Cravings

The more you are deprived of something, the more your body craves it. Only time can heal this problem. Thus, we stress that you need to have strong willpower to control your cravings.

Coconut Oil Fried Veggies and Eggs

This recipe will never bore you. It keeps you full for a very long time so you won't crave a mini burger every two hours!

SERVES: 2
PREPARATION TIME: 15 min
INGREDIENTS:
Coconut oil 2 tablespoons
Spinach 1 cup
Frozen mixed vegetables 1-2 cups
Salt ½ teaspoon
Pepper ¼ teaspoon
Eggs 3-4
METHOD:

1. Thaw the frozen vegetables.
2. Preheat the frying pan and pour in the coconut oil.
3. Add thawed vegetables. Stir well.
4. Whisk eggs and add to the frying pan. Stir well.
5. Sprinkle salt and pepper on the vegetables.
6. Add chopped spinach to the mixture. Stir properly with the eggs. Stir fry the mixture until the eggs are ready.

Grilled Chicken Wings with Salsa and Veg

Chicken is always tasty, no matter what form you get it in. The salsa sauce and a mix of spices make this dish special.

SERVES: 2-3

PREPARATION TIME: 15 min for preparation, 1 hour for baking and refrigerating

INGREDIENTS:

Chicken wings 500 grams
Spice mix 2-3 teaspoons
Cauliflower ½ cup
Bell peppers ½ cup
Beans ¼ cup
Cucumber ½ cup
Tomato ½ cup
Salsa 3 tablespoons
Salt 1.5 teaspoons
Pepper 1 teaspoon

METHOD:

1. Marinate the chicken wings by sprinkling the spice mix on them.
2. Preheat the oven to 180-200 degrees.
3. Once oven has heated, put the chicken into the oven for approximately 40 minutes.
4. You must grill the wings till they become crunchy and brown.
5. Take a skillet and stir-fry the chopped vegetables- cauliflower, bell pepper, beans, cucumber, and tomato. Cook them till crisp.
6. Sprinkle salt and pepper over the vegetables.
7. Take them off the heat and let them cool.
8. You can also refrigerate the vegetables if you like for an hour. Take the chicken out of the oven and serve hot with chilled vegetables and salsa.

Eggs and Bacon

Though bacon is a processed meat, it is low in carbohydrate content. Thus, you can consume it once or twice a week if you want to lose weight. Besides, it tastes good!

SERVES: 2
PREPARATION TIME: 15 min
INGREDIENTS:
Bacon 8 ounces
Eggs 3-4
Garlic powder ½ teaspoon
Onion powder ½ teaspoon
Spice mix 1 teaspoon
Sea salt ½ teaspoon
Pepper ¼ teaspoon
METHOD:

1. Preheat a pan and pour in a teaspoon of coconut oil.
2. Put in bacon and stir-fry until it becomes tender.
3. Sprinkle spice mix, onion powder and garlic powder onto bacon and mix.
4. Take the bacon out on a plate when ready.
5. Scramble the eggs and stir-fry in the bacon fat. Add sea salt and pepper and mix well till cooked through.
6. Serve hot on plate with bacon.

Ground Beef & Bell Peppers

This is a delicious beef meal that you can eat whenever you want. Take any leftovers to work in your lunchbox the next day.

SERVES: 2
PREPARATION TIME: 15 min
INGREDIENTS:

Coconut oil 2 teaspoons
Ground beef 5-6 ounces
Sliced Onions 1-2 medium
Red chili ½ teaspoon
Coriander ¼ teaspoon
Bay leaves 2
Clove powder ¼ teaspoon
Cinnamon powder ¼ teaspoon
Sliced bell peppers 1
Spinach ½ cup

METHOD:

1. Preheat a frying pan and pour coconut oil into it.
2. Put in the bay leaves and stir.
3. Put the sliced onions into the oil and sauté.
4. Add ground beef to the pan and stir.
5. Add the spices (red chili, coriander, clove powder and cinnamon powder) to the mixture and mix well.
6. Add spinach.
7. Cook until beef becomes tender. Place on a serving plate.

8. Put sliced bell peppers into the remaining oil in the frying pan and sauté for a minute or so.
9. Serve on top of the beef.

Low-Carb No Bun Cheeseburgers

This recipe is low on carbohydrate intake because there is no grain-bun used in the dish. The melted cheese on the top is a delicious treat. It is difficult to get bored with this amazing mouth-watering cheeseburger.

SERVES: 2
PREPARATION TIME: 15 min
INGREDIENTS:
Butter 2 tablespoons
Frozen Hamburgers 2
Cheddar cheese 1 tablespoon
Cream cheese 1 tablespoon
Salsa 2 tablespoon
Spice mix 1-2 teaspoons
Spinach ½ cup
METHOD:

1. Preheat a frying pan and put some butter in it.
2. Put two burgers in the butter and fry them for 2-3 minutes or until they are brown.
3. Flip them over and fry from on the other side too.
4. When they are light brown in color, put the spice mix on the burgers.
5. Add some cheddar cheese slices and some chunks of cream cheese. Do not stir.
6. Turn down the flame or heat and let the cheese melt.
7. Take the hamburgers out on a plate and serve them with shredded spinach.
8. Pour some of the fat left in the frying pan over the spinach as well as a dressing.
9. Top the burgers with salsa to make them even juicier.

Fried Chicken Breasts

Chicken breasts are so juicy and yummy that they can be had anytime of the day. You do not have to think twice before making this quick dish.

SERVES: 2
PREPARATION TIME: 15 min
INGREDIENTS:
Butter 2 tablespoons
Chicken breasts 6-8 ounces
Salt 2 teaspoons
Pepper 1 teaspoon
Garlic powder ½ teaspoon
Curry powder ½ teaspoon
Vegetables (bell pepper and onions) ½ cup

METHOD:

1. Cut the chicken breasts into small pieces.
2. Preheat a pan and add butter to it.
3. Add the pieces of chicken to the frying pan.
4. Add spices to the chicken- garlic powder, salt, pepper and curry.
5. Stir fry the chicken until it turns brown. You will notice a crunchy texture in the meat after a while.
6. Place it on a plate.
7. Put the sliced bell peppers and onions in the pan and sauté for 30 seconds.
8. Take the vegetables out and serve them with the chicken.
9. The chicken is already juicy in texture. So there is no need to add any sauce. Still, if you feel that it is dry, you can serve some salsa sauce along with it.

Fake Meat Pizza

You might have been missing pizza after switching to the ketogenic diet. Here we have a healthy solution for you. This meat-za is prepared with absolutely healthy ingredients with all the familiar flavors of a pizza. Moreover, you can modify this versatile recipe with as many ingredients as you want. Just indulge into it without any guilt.

SERVES: 2
PREPARATION TIME: 15 min
BAKING TIME: 40 min
INGREDIENTS:

Ground beef 5 ounces
Salsa 2-3 tablespoons
Onions 2-3 medium
Garlic powder 2 teaspoons
Shredded cheese ½ cup
Bacon 10-15 pieces
Spice mix 2 teaspoons

METHOD:

1. Preheat the oven to 180-200 degrees.
2. Meanwhile, dice the onions and bacon.
3. Mix the onions, ground beef, salsa, garlic powder and spice mix in a bowl. Press onto the bottom of a greased round baking dish.
4. Put some shredded cheese on top of the mixture.
5. Spread the slices of bacon over the top.
6. Put the baking dish into the oven for 30-40 minutes or until the cheese and bacon look crunchy.
7. Take out the dish and serve wedges of this meat-za on a plate.

Cheesy Egg & Bacon

If you make this delicious egg and bacon just once, you'll make it over and over again. Don't worry, though- all the ingredients are good for you!

SERVES: 2
PREPARATION TIME: 15 min
INGREDIENTS:

Eggs 6
Milk 1 cup
Melted butter 2 tablespoons
Chopped spring onions ¼ cup
Chopped bacon rashers 5
Grated cheese 1 cup
Chopped Cilantro ¼ cup

METHOD:

1. Preheat the oven to 180 degrees.
2. Take a frying pan and sauté bacon to render out the excess fat.
3. Take a medium sized bowl and whisk the eggs with butter and milk.
4. Season the mixture with pepper and salt.
5. Take a rectangular baking dish and pour the egg mixture into it.
6. Spread bacon rashers and cheese onto the dish. Sprinkle onions over evenly.
7. Put the baking dish in the oven and cook for 30-40 minutes. When the egg sets in the middle, remove from the oven.
8. Cut into portions and serve garnished with green cilantro.
9. May be served with a side of green salad.

Spicy Shrimp & Mashed Cauliflower

Shrimps are the perfect warm food for those cold autumn months. Moreover, in this recipe, you learn a substitute for starchy potatoes. We are giving you a recipe for cauliflower starch, which looks like mashed potato, tastes like mashed potato and satisfies your craving for starch like mashed potato does. When you are getting all the benefits of potatoes from cauliflower, then you can think about completely quitting potatoes.

SERVES: 2
PREPARATION TIME: 15 min
INGREDIENTS (for cauliflower mash):
Cauliflower florets 4 cups
Mayonnaise 1/3 cup
Peeled and minced garlic 1 clove
Water 1 tablespoon
Kosher salt 1 teaspoon
Black pepper 1/8 teaspoon
Lemon juice ¼ teaspoon
Lemon zest ½ teaspoon
Fresh chopped chives 1 tablespoon
INGREDIENTS (for shrimps):
Frozen shrimps 16 ounce
Butter 2 tablespoons
Salt 1 teaspoon
Pepper ½ teaspoon
Sriracha chili sauce 2 tablespoons

METHOD (for cauliflower mash):

1. Take a large microwave-safe bowl and mix the mayonnaise, cauliflower, water, garlic, pepper and salt.
2. Microwave the mixture on high for nearly 12-15 minutes.
3. When the mixture becomes very soft, mash it with a potato masher if you like a coarse texture.
4. If you prefer a smooth texture, puree the mixture with a blender.
5. Add lemon juice, lemon zest and chives. Mix them well. Serve warm.

METHOD (for shrimps):

1. Take a large sauce pan and heat it over medium-high heat.
2. Put butter into it and let it melt.
3. Peel and thaw the shrimp. Toss into the pan and sauté.
4. Cook for about 4-6 minutes until the shrimps become pink.
5. Add salt and pepper to the shrimps and mix well.
6. Add the sriracha sauce and mix in. If you want a spicy dish, add more than 2 tablespoons of sauce.
7. Cook for another 2 minutes and then remove the pan from the heat.
8. Place some cauliflower mash in a plate and top it with shrimps. Enjoy!

Bacon & Brussels Sprouts

While Brussels sprouts aren't a complete dish on their own, you just need to add shallots, bacon and garlic to make a tasty main or side dish.

SERVES: 2
PREPARATION TIME: 15 min
INGREDIENTS:

Chopped bacon (center cut) 6 slices
Sliced shallots ½ cup
Brussels sprouts 1.5 pounds
Thinly sliced garlic cloves 6
Fat free chicken broth (lower sodium) ¾ cup
Salt 1/8 teaspoon
Black pepper (freshly ground) 1/8 teaspoon

METHOD:

1. Take a large skillet and heat it over medium heat.
2. Put bacon in, and cook for 5 minutes till brown.
3. Remove the pan from the heat.
4. Take out the bacon with a deep spoon.
5. Keep 1 tablespoon of dripping in the skillet and discard the rest.
6. Put the skillet back on the heat and put in bacon, Brussels sprouts and shallot. Sauté together for 4 minutes.
7. Add garlic and stir together for a few minutes.
8. Add chicken broth and let it boil.
9. Stirring now and then allow the broth to almost evaporate (takes about 2 minutes). The sprouts will become crisp-tender.
10. Sprinkle with pepper and salt and remove from heat.
11. Serve hot.

Easy & Quick Tomato Soup

Just look around your kitchen and refrigerator. You might find that you already have the ingredients for this quick and creamy soup recipe. This is a warming and healthy soup.

SERVES: 3
PREPARATION TIME: 15 min
INGREDIENTS:

Butter 2 tablespoons
Onions ½ cup
Undrained diced tomatoes 1 can of 28 ounces
Chicken broth 2 cups
Heavy cream 1 cup
Salt ½ teaspoon
Pepper ¼ teaspoon
Minced parsley 2 tablespoons

METHOD:

1. Take a deep saucepan and heat it over a medium-high heat.
2. Put in the butter and let it melt.
3. Add onions and sauté them until they become tender.
4. Add tomatoes along with their liquid into the pan. Mix well and let the mixture boil.
5. Simmer on low heat for 5 minutes.
6. Turn off the heat and puree the mixture with a hand blender.
7. Add the cream and stir well.
8. Add seasoning and mix in.
9. Add parsley and serve hot.

Salami with Goat Cheese

Delicious rolls of rich salami combined with fresh arugula make a lovely dish for an afternoon meal. Not only they are carbohydrate free, they will keep you satiated for many hours. Moreover, the arugula in the rolls lowers high blood pressure and reduces the amount of oxygen a person needs during a work-out. It has also been proven to enhance performance during athletics.

SERVES: 5
PREPARATION TIME: 15 min
INGREDIENTS:
Genoa salami (thin slices) 14 slices or 3.5 ounces
Goat cheese (fresh) 3 ounces
Baby arugula 2 ounces
Olive oil (extra virgin) 1 tablespoon
Vinegar (red wine) 2 teaspoons
Kosher salt ½ teaspoon
Pepper ¼ teaspoon
METHOD:

1. On a large tray, arrange the slices of salami in one layer.
2. Spoon a small heap of goats cheese in the middle of every slice.
3. Take a bowl and mix the arugula with vinegar and olive oil.
4. Season with pepper and salt.
5. Divide the arugula mixture onto all the salami slices. Roll the slices.
6. Cut the rolls in half. When you want to serve them, keep the seam down on the platter to prevent their opening, or tie up with chive leaves as illustrated.

Stuffed Deviled Eggs

These deviled eggs are ideal for kids' birthday parties. Not only they are quick to prepare, they are awesome to eat as well. If your kids find them too spicy, you can adjust the amounts of mayonnaise and mustard. You can also serve them to the adults garnished with finely chopped chives or parsley and paprika.

SERVES: 4
PREPARATION TIME: 15 min
COOKING TIME: 30 min
INGREDIENTS:

Eggs 12
Mayonnaise 2 tablespoons
Chinese mustard 1 teaspoon
Yellow mustard 2 teaspoons
Salt as per taste
Pepper as per taste
Paprika ½ teaspoon
Chopped chives 1 tablespoon

METHOD:

1. Take a large saucepan and place all the eggs in it.
2. Cover them with water and bring it to boil.
3. Remove the pan from the heat and cover it with a lid.
4. Let the eggs stand in the hot water for 10-12 minutes.
5. Remove the eggs from the water. Let them cool and then peel.
6. Slice the eggs lengthwise in half. Remove the yolks.
7. Put the yolks in a bowl and add mayonnaise.
8. Mash them with yellow mustard, Chinese mustard, pepper

and salt.
9. Fill the egg whites which you hollowed earlier with this mixture of egg yolks. You can use a teaspoon or piping bag.
10. Sprinkle with paprika and chopped chives to garnish.
11. Refrigerate these eggs until you serve them.

Low Carb Chili Beef in Rich Tomato Gravy

This recipe takes a long cooking time but it is worth it. The preparation takes only 15 minutes. You will go back to this recipe again and again once you serve it to your family. The rich flavor of the tomato gravy is absolutely delicious.

SERVES: 4
PREPARATION TIME: 15 min
COOKING TIME: 2 hours simmer cook
INGREDIENTS:
Ground beef 1.25 pounds
Tomato paste 8 ounce
Chopped tomatoes 1.5
Chopped red bell pepper 1
Chopped onion ½ cup
Chopped celery sticks 2
Cumin seeds 1.5 teaspoons
Chili powder 1 teaspoon
Pepper ½ teaspoon
Salt 1 teaspoon
Water ¾ cup or more if needed

METHOD:

1. Preheat a medium-sized pan and put ground beef into it.
2. Cook until it becomes brown.
3. Add the onions along with bell peppers and sauté them with

beef for 1-2 minutes.
4. Take a medium or large pot and combine onions, cooked meat, tomatoes, peppers, tomato paste, celery and water.
5. Sprinkle all the spices into the pot. Bring the ingredients to boil and then simmer on low heat for 1-2 hours. Stir every 30 minutes.
6. Serve hot.

Keto Quick Gravy

It takes hardly any time to prepare this gravy. It is very delicious for a complete meal at the breakfast table. The breakfast sausages absolutely complement the gravy. You can have this dish as a complete meal in itself or you can also have it as a side dish with burgers and salami sandwiches.

SERVES: 5
PREPARATION TIME: 10 min
INGREDIENTS:

Breakfast sausage 4 ounce
Butter 2 tablespoon
Heavy cream 1 cup
Guar gum powder ½ teaspoon
Salt as per taste
Pepper as per taste
Cilantro for garnishing

METHOD:

1. Take a large saucepan and heat it on medium-high heat.
2. Put the breakfast sausages in the pan and cook them until they become brown.
3. Take the sausages out with a deep spoon and leave the fat behind.
4. Put the butter into the pan and melt it.
5. Add heavy cream when the butter is melted. Stir when the bubbles are formed.
6. Put guar gum powder into the cream. Stir vigorously to burst the bubbles.
7. When the mixture becomes thick, you will notice that the gap left from stirring takes a while to fill in with gravy.
8. Put the sausages back into the pan and stir.
9. Serve hot.

Southern Spicy Chicken Salad

This is an amazingly simple chicken salad which uses up your leftover chicken and can be served with tomato wedges and pickles all piled onto a bed of lettuce for a quick fresh summer lunch.

SERVES: 5
PREPARATION TIME: 10 min
INGREDIENTS:
Cooked and chopped chicken 10-12 ounces
Butter 2 tablespoons
Red onion (finely chopped) 3 tablespoons
Celery (finely chopped) 2-3 tablespoons
Chopped hard-boiled egg 1 large
Dill pickle 1 tablespoon
Mayonnaise ½ cup
Salt ¼ teaspoon
Black pepper (freshly ground) 1/8 teaspoon

METHOD:

1. Take a medium sized sauté pan and heat it on medium high heat.
2. Melt the butter in the pan and put the chicken pieces into it.
3. Cook the chicken until it becomes brown.
4. Take it off the heat.
5. Take a medium-sized bowl and combine onions, chicken, eggs, and celery and toss them together.
6. Add the dill pickle, salt, mayonnaise, pepper and mix well.
7. Serve garnished with raw tomatoes and chopped mint leaves on a bed of lettuce.

Keto Spinach Soup

This soup is a superfood that you can never underestimate. All its ingredients are rich in nutrients. It gives you an ample supply of antioxidants, magnesium, potassium and lots of vitamins. It also gives you an ample amount of calcium without using any dairy products.
This will help kick off your "ketogeinc flu" which sometimes overcomes new followers of this diet.

SERVES: 5
PREPARATION TIME: 10 min
INGREDIENTS:
Cauliflower (medium head) 1 or 400 grams
White onion (medium) 1
Garlic cloves 2
Crumbled bay leaf 1
Watercress 150 grams
Fresh spinach 200 grams
Vegetable or chicken stock 1 liter
Coconut milk or cream 1 cup
Coconut oil ¼ cup
Salt 1 teaspoon
Black pepper (freshly ground) ½ teaspoon
Chives/Parsley for garnishing

METHOD:

1. Take a deep saucepan and put the coconut oil into it. When the oil is heated over medium heat, put in finely chopped garlic and onions. Sauté until the vegetables become tender.
2. Wash the watercress and spinach and keep aside.
3. Cut the florets of cauliflower and combine them with the onions.
4. Add the bay leaf and mix the ingredients well.
5. Add watercress and spinach leaves. Cook for 2-3 minutes until leaves are wilted.
6. Pour the in chicken or vegetable stock. Bring the mixture to a boil.
7. When the cauliflower becomes crisp-tender, pour in the coconut milk or cream.
8. Sprinkle with pepper and salt and mix well.
9. Take the saucepan off the heat and puree with a hand blender.
10. When the mixture is a nice creamy texture, it's ready to serve.
11. Pour some cream over the soup in the bowl just before serving.
12. Garnish with chives or parsley leaves.

Orange Coconut Drink

If you have to rush to the office on a Monday morning after a long weekend party, just wait for a second. Take just 10 minutes before you rush out and make this awesome and satisfying smoothie. It tastes amazing and will keep you energized for hours. Orange is not only good for your skin; it takes care of your heart as well.

SERVES: 4
PREPARATION TIME: 10 min
INGREDIENTS:
Orange juice 4 cups
Ice 2 cups
Coconut milk 1 can of ½ ounces
Honey ¼ cup
Shredded coconut 2 tablespoons
Orange slices for garnish

METHOD:

1. Put the coconut milk, orange juice, honey and ice into a large jug and blend using a hand blender.
2. Puree until the mixture becomes very smooth.
3. You can also make it less smooth if you prefer a coarse texture.
4. Pour the smoothie into four glasses and garnish with orange slices and shredded coconut.

Salmon Spread

You can get as creative with serving this salmon spread as you want to be. Serve it as a dip or with a salad of tomatoes, cucumbers, bell peppers, etc. You can also use it as a filling for mushroom caps and serve it in a ready eat format at a get together.

It takes just 10 minutes to make then refrigerate it for an upcoming party.

SERVES: 5
PREPARATION TIME: 10 min
INGREDIENTS:

Cream cheese 12 ounces
Sour cream 1/3 cup
Lemon juice, fresh 1 tablespoon
Tabasco sauce 6 dashes
Green and white parts of scallions 3
Drained and rinsed capers 3 tablespoons
Coarsely chopped smoked salmon 8 ounces
Fresh dill 3 tablespoons

METHOD:

1. Put sour cream, cream cheese, Tabasco and lemon juice in a food processor and pulse till they become a puree.
2. Add the capers, scallions, salmon, pepper and chopped dill. Blend them with the rest of the puree.
3. Take the puree out of the blender.
4. You can use this salmon spread with burgers, lettuce sandwiches, etc. You can also spread a mound of this salmon spread over chilled cucumber slices and serve it as a salad.

Fried Eggs With Cheddar Garlic and Cooking Grits

A quick recipe for a delicious breakfast. This will fill you up till lunchtime!

SERVES: 5
PREPARATION TIME: 10 min
INGREDIENTS:

Water 2 cups
Cooking grits ½ cup
Grated garlic clove 1
Cheddar cheese, grated ¼ cup
Chopped chives 1 tablespoon
Large eggs 4
Salt and pepper as per taste
Butter ½ teaspoon

METHOD:

1. Pour water into a small saucepan and bring it to boil.
2. When the water boils, reduce the heat to simmer or medium.
3. Put garlic and cooking grits in the pan and stir. Cover the pan with a lid.
4. Cook and stir frequently for 5-7 minutes until you find that the cooking grits are thickened.
5. Take the pan off the heat and add chives and grated cheddar cheese. Combine the ingredients well.
6. Add pepper and salt as per your taste. Keep the mixture aside.
7. Take a non-stick frying pan and heat it over medium heat.
8. Put some butter to grease the pan and crack the eggs in the frying pan. You can crack two eggs at a time.
9. Cook until the egg whites turn opaque.
10. Flip the eggs over and cook for a while.
11. Pour the cooking grits into shallow bowls and top with the eggs. Season with salt and pepper.

12. Serve immediately and piping hot.

Cup Omelets

Eggs are one thing which can be given any shape, size and look. You can add virtually anything to eggs and the outcome will be probably be good. Here, we have experimented to give eggs a new shape and added some vegetables. This is a perfect afternoon meal.

SERVES: 6
PREPARATION TIME: 10 min
BAKING TIME: 25 min
INGREDIENTS:

Eggs 4
Salt as per taste
Pepper as per taste
Diced bell pepper ½ cup
Diced tomato ½ cup
Diced cucumber ½ cup
Diced onions ½ cup
Shredded cheese ¾ cup
Chopped cilantro for garnishing

METHOD:

1. Preheat the oven to at least 350 degrees.
2. Take a muffin pan with six cups and coat it with a cooking spray (nonstick).
3. Mix all the vegetables in a skillet and sauté them for 30 seconds.
4. Whisk all the eggs in a medium sized bowl.
5. Add diced vegetables to the bowl.
6. Add salt and pepper according to your taste.
7. Share out the mixture among the muffin cups and sprinkle

shredded cheese over the top.
8. Put the muffin tray in the oven and bake for about 20-25 minutes. The edges of the omelets will become golden brown.
9. When you are about to remove the omelets from the cups, run a blunt butter knife around the cup edges to loosen.
10. Take out the omelet cups in a plate and garnish with a little cilantro.
11. Serve hot.

Tomato Scoops filled with Avocado

Little tomato halves stuffed with gorgeous creamy avocado. These make a delicious and colorful snack for any time of the day.

SERVES: 3-4
PREPARATION TIME: 15 min
INGREDIENTS:

Cherry tomatoes 16 ounces
Mashed and peeled avocado 1 large
Lemon juice 1 tablespoon
Onion (finely chopped) 1
Minced garlic 1 clove
Swiss cheese (finely shredded) ½ cup
Seasoning salt ¼ teaspoon
Bacon bits (bottled) 6 slices

METHOD:

1. Remove the top green part of the tomatoes. Cut about 1/3 part of the tomatoes.
2. Take a deep spoon and scoop out the seeds. Keep them for use in another dish. They will not be used in this recipe again.
3. Place the tomatoes on a paper towel with the cut-side facing downwards.
4. Cut the avocado and remove its pit.
5. Scoop out the flesh into a bowl and add seasoning salt and lemon juice.
6. Mash all the ingredients in the bowl using a fork. You can keep the mixture a little coarse.
7. Stuff the mixture of avocado into the tomato scoops.
8. Sprinkle some bacon bits on top and serve.

White Bean Salmon Salad

This delicious and filling salad makes a perfect light lunch or supper dish. The simple dressing compliments it perfectly, and as a bonus, the whole thing packs and keeps well in a lunchbox for work or school.

SERVES: 3-4
PREPARATION TIME: 15 min
INGREDIENTS FOR SALAD:

Cannellini beans 2 cans (15 ounces each)
Pink salmon 1 can (3.75 ounces)
Parmesan cheese (freshly grated) ¼ cup
Red onion, minced ¼ cup
Minced garlic 1 clove
Tomatoes (cut into 8 pieces each) 2
Roughly chopped basil leaves ¼ cup

INGREDIENTS FOR DRESSING:

Vinegar 3 tablespoons
Olive oil, extra virgin ¼ cup
Coarse salt ¼ teaspoon
Ground pepper 1/8 teaspoon

METHOD:

1. Remove beans from can, drain, and put them in a bowl.
2. Flake the salmon over the beans. Grate the parmesan cheese and sprinkle over the mixture.
3. Add the basil leaves, onions, tomatoes and minced garlic to the bowl.
4. Whisk the ingredients of the dressing together and pour it over the mixture of beans.
5. Gently toss the ingredients in the bowl and combine well.
6. Refrigerate the salad for 15 minutes and serve.

Chicken Lettuce Burrito

Do you miss your regular tortillas? Now you don't have to. The delicious lettuce rolls mentioned in the recipe will never let you say that you "can't eat those rolls anymore". You can have these lettuce rolls as much as you want without worrying about the side effects of wheat.

SERVES: 3-4
PREPARATION TIME: 15-20 min
INGREDIENTS:
Chicken breast (boneless halves) 2 (skinless)
Tomato sauce 1 can (4 ounces)
Salsa ¼ cup
Diced bell peppers 1
Chopped beans ½ cup
Taco seasoning mix 1.25 ounces
Ground cumin 1 teaspoon
Minced garlic 2 cloves
Chili powder 1 teaspoon
Hot sauce as per taste
Large lettuce leaves 8-10

METHOD:

1. Take a medium saucepan and heat it over medium heat.
2. Place tomato sauce and chicken breasts in the pan and cook until the sauce comes to boil.
3. Add salsa, cumin, garlic, chili powder and seasoning to the pan.
4. Simmer it for 15 minutes.
5. You can add a little water if you find that the mixture has become very thick.
6. Using 2 forks shred and pull the chicken meat off the main chunk into thin strings.
7. Add the bell peppers and beans to the pot.
8. Cook the strings and vegetables with lid on for another 8-10 minutes.
9. Add hot sauce as per your taste. Stir well.
10. When you find that the mixture has attained a thick consistency that can be easily wrapped, take it off the heat.
11. Place two layers of lettuce on a tray and fill it up with the filling.
12. Serve hot.

Shrimp Skewers and Lime Honey Dipping Sauce

Grilled shrimps are always good in summer. And what's better is when they are accompanied by a lime honey sauce. The freshness of the shrimps is retained even after cooking. They are just as good as they can get for a ketogenic diet. Indulge in this satisfying dish and enjoy the sunny day lunch.

SERVES: 3-4
PREPARATION TIME: 15 min
INGREDIENTS (for shrimps):

Peeled shrimps 1 pound
Salt 1 teaspoon
Pepper ½ teaspoon
Garlic powder ½ teaspoon
Skewers 3-4

INGREDIENTS (for lime honey sauce):

Olive oil 1 tablespoon
Honey 3 full tablespoons
Limes for juice 2 large
Lemon zest 1 lemon
Chili powder ½ teaspoon
Cilantro ½ cup

METHOD (for shrimps):

1. Preheat a grill frying pan over a medium heat.
2. Spray the non-stick cooking spray around the pan.
3. Place the shrimps onto the skewers
4. Mix the pepper, salt and garlic powder and sprinkle the

mixture over the shrimps.

METHOD (for sauce):

1. Take a small bowl and mix the honey, olive oil, chili powder, lime juice and lemon zest.
2. Take out 2 tablespoons of this mixture and brush the shrimps with it.
3. Keep the remaining sauce for serving.
4. After brushing the shrimps, grill them for 3-4 minutes.
5. After one side is cooked properly, flip them over and cook for 3-4 minutes.
6. When properly cooked the shrimps should look pinkish in color.
7. Take them off the heat. Place them in a plate and sprinkle some cilantro over them.
8. Serve with the lime honey sauce.

Zucchini Wraps

If you missed eating wraps in the ketogenic diet, here we are, with a beautiful option. These zucchini wraps are a completely healthy substitute for those refined flour wraps.
They are spread with a fresh-tasting pesto, then layered with vegetable strips before being rolled up.

SERVES: 2
PREPARATION TIME: 15 min
INGREDIENTS (for wraps):
Thinly sliced zucchini (lengthwise) 3
Julienned bell pepper (red) 1
Julienned bell pepper (yellow) 1
Julienned quarters of carrots 1 carrot
Sprouts as per choice
Cilantro ¼ cup
Freshly ground black pepper ¼ teaspoon
Toothpicks 7-8

INGREDIENTS (for kale pesto):
Basil leaves or kale 1 cup
Garlic 1 clove
Tahini 2 tablespoons
Olive oil, extra virgin 2 tablespoons
Himalayan salt as per taste

METHOD:

1. For making the kale pesto, put the kale or basil leaves, garlic, tahini, olive oil and Himalayan salt into a food processor and pulse.
2. Add more seasoning if you feel it is needed.
3. Layer the zucchini slices on a chopping board. Layer on the pesto, bell peppers, carrots and sprouts. Roll the zucchini picking up the end where the vegetables are placed.
4. Stick the zucchini rolls with a toothpick in the middle. Sprinkle some freshly ground black pepper over the rolls.
5. Serve.

Eggs and Kale Blessing

Kale is a relatively new introduction to the American platter. But, it is the most nutrient dense vegetable of the cruciferous vegetable family. The high content of antioxidants in this leafy vegetable is not found anywhere else. Thus, it is ideal to include in a quick and healthy evening snack or an early morning breakfast.

SERVES: 1
PREPARATION TIME: 15 min
INGREDIENTS:
Butter 4 tablespoons
Minced garlic 1 clove
Kale ½ pound
Eggs 2
Coconut cream 1 tablespoon
Salt 1 pinch
Freshly ground black pepper ¼ teaspoon
METHOD (for kale and eggs):

1. Take a small skillet and melt the butter in it over medium heat.
2. Add the minced garlic to the skillet. Cook it for a minute.
3. While the garlic cooks, trim the baby kale leaves from stems and wash them. Add them to the skillet.
4. Cover the skillet and let the baby kale cook for 5 minutes until wilted.
5. Remove from the skillet and keep warm.
6. Separate one of the eggs into yolk and white. Put in separate bowls.
7. Add one complete egg into the bowl containing only egg

white.
8. Add one more tablespoon of butter into the skillet. Pour in the egg white mixture and cook until the egg white turns opaque.

METHOD (for sauce):

1. Microwave the coconut cream (1 tablespoon) and butter (2 tablespoons) just enough to melt them.
2. In the food processor, put a dash of salt, egg yolk (which we had separated earlier) and freshly ground black pepper.
3. Pulse the mixture and slowly pour the coconut cream and butter mix. Pulse the mixture till you have a smooth cream.

METHOD (for serving):

When ready to serve, place the kale in a plate. Place the fried egg over the kale. Spoon over as much sauce as you like.

Shrimp, Avocado and Spinach Salad with Lemon Zest Dressing

A lovely satisfying salad that serves as a light lunch or dinner. A bed of baby spinach topped with avocado, tomato and cucumber, shrimps, and dressed to perfection with a lemony dressing.

SERVES: 3-4
PREPARATION TIME: 15 min
INGREDIENTS:

Avocado 1
Baby spinach 5 ounces
Garlic 1 clove
Cherry tomatoes/ normal tomatoes ½ pint
Cucumber slices 8-10
Lemon juice 1 teaspoon
Lemon zest ½ lemon
Peeled shrimp ½ pound
Coconut oil 1 tablespoon

METHOD:

1. Wash the spinach and dry it on a paper towel.
2. Wash the cherry tomatoes and cut them into half. If you are using normal tomatoes, cut them into 8 wedges.
3. Halve the avocado and remove the pit. Scoop out the flesh with a melon baller.
4. Wash the shrimps under cold water and dry them on a paper towel.
5. Preheat a medium skillet.
6. Add the coconut oil to the skillet. Swirl the skillet so that the oil coats the bottom of the pan entirely.
7. Add garlic and let it cook until a gentle fragrance starts coming.

8. Add shrimps to the skillet and cook for 1-2 minutes on each side. The shrimps will become opaque when properly cooked.
9. To prepare the dressing, take a small bowl and put in the olive oil, lemon juice, lemon zest, honey, pepper and salt. Combine them together.
10. Arrange a layer of spinach on a plate. Put the avocado, tomatoes, cucumber slices and shrimps over the spinach. Pour some dressing and serve.

Flour Free Cheese Crackers

Sometimes, you just feel like munching something without any reason. For such cravings, we often resort to biscuits. Since it is better that you do not eat anything made of flour in the ketogenic diet; we have devised these cheese crackers for you. They will come in handy for those peckish moments when you want something crunchy to munch.

SERVES: 4
PREPARATION TIME: 15 min
INGREDIENTS:
Cheese 8 ounces
Parchment paper for lining a baking dish
Seasoning ½ teaspoon
Mayonnaise for serving
METHOD:

1. Preheat your oven to a temperature of 400 degrees.
2. Take a medium-sized baking sheet and line it with a parchment paper.
3. You can follow either one of two methods:

Shred cheese in a bowl and add some seasonings. "or"
Cut the cheese into thin slices and sprinkle with seasoning.

1. Put tablespoons of shredded cheese onto the parchment. If you have cut slices (1/4 inch thickness) of cheese, place them on the parchment paper.
2. Leave a gap of 1 inch in between the cheese slices or piles.
3. Put the baking sheet into the oven and cook for 5-7 minutes.
4. You will notice that the edges of cheese will become brown when properly cooked.
5. Take out the baking dish and allow it to cool.

6. The cheese crackers will become crispy as they cool.
7. Serve them at room temperature later with mayonnaise or any other dip you like.

Bok Choy and Crispy Tofu Salad

This is a delicious recipe for tofu salad. The preparation does not take much time, but you do need to allow for some extra time for the marinating. Ultimately, the end result is of course worth it. You just need to plan ahead a little.

SERVES: 4
PREPARATION TIME: 25 min
MARINATING TIME: 5-6 hours
INGREDIENTS (tofu):
Firm tofu 15 ounces
Soy sauce 1 tablespoon
Sesame oil 1 tablespoon
Water 1 tablespoon
Minced garlic 2 teaspoons
Red wine vinegar 1 tablespoon
Lemon juice 1 teaspoon
INGREDIENTS (salad):
Bok choy 9 ounces
Green onion 2.5 ounces
Chopped cilantro 2 tablespoons
Coconut oil 3 tablespoons
Soy sauce 2 tablespoons
Sambal oelek (sauce) 1 tablespoon
Peanut butter 1 tablespoon
Lime juice 1 teaspoon
Liquid stevia 7 drops
METHOD:

1. Press the tofu dry for about 5-6 hours before cooking.

2. To prepare the marinade, combine the soy sauce, water, sesame oil, lemon juice, vinegar and garlic.
3. Make small dices of tofu and marinate them in the mixture for at least 30 minutes. It is better if you leave it to marinate for 5-6 hours.
4. Preheat your oven to 350 degrees.
5. Take a medium-sized baking sheet and line it with parchment paper.
6. Place the marinated tofu onto the baking sheet and cook for 30-35 minutes.
7. While the tofu is baking, take a bowl and combine all the ingredients for the salad dressing, leaving the bok choy aside.
8. Chop the bok choy into small pieces.
9. Remove the tofu from the oven.
10. Arrange the tofu, bok choy and salad dressing on a plate and serve.

Zucchini Pasta and Basil-Cashew Pesto

Did you think that you would not be able to have all those delicious pastas when you're are on a keto diet? Well, it is better that you say goodbye to those unhealthy refined flour pastas. We have a much healthier option for you. It's zucchini pasta! The pesto sauce along with this green vegetable is so tasty.

SERVES: 2
PREPARATION TIME: 15 min
INGREDIENTS:
Basil leaves ½ cup
Minced garlic 2 cloves
Cashew nuts (raw) ¼ cup
Olive oil (extra virgin) ¼ cup
Lime juice 1 tablespoons
Nutritional yeast 1.5 tablespoons
Zucchini 2
Salt ½ teaspoon
METHOD:

1. Put the basil leaves, garlic, cashew nuts, olive oil, lime juice and yeast in a food processor and pulse to make the pesto.
2. Using a spiralizer, make noodles out of the zucchini.
3. Take a skillet and sauté zucchini pasta.
4. Remove the pasta from the skillet and put it into a bowl.
5. Remove the pesto from the food processor and mix it with the pasta.
6. Serve with a smile.

Cheese Broccoli Soup
SERVES: 2
PREPARATION TIME: 15 min
INGREDIENTS:

Pastured butter 2 tablespoons
Chicken broth 3 cups
Organic cream cheese 8 ounces
Heavy cream 1 cup
Cheddar cheese, shredded 2 cups
Chopped fresh broccoli 2 bunches

METHOD:

1. Take a deep saucepan and put the chicken broth and broccoli into it.
2. Bring to the boil and cook until the broccoli becomes tender.
3. Take a frying pan and put it on the heat.
4. Put in the heavy cream, shredded cheese, cream cheese, and butter. Stir well.
5. Take half of the broccoli from the pot and puree it in a food processor.
6. Pour the melted mixture from the pan into the saucepan of broth. Put the pureed broccoli from the food processor into the broth as well.
7. Combine well. Add pepper and salt according to taste.
8. When you feel that the soup has reached a desired thickness and is a good consistency, ladle into soup bowls.
9. Garnish with cheese.
10. Serve hot.

Avocado Wrapped in Bacon

Creamy avocado with salty bacon! Sounds delicious doesn't it? These bites of bacon wrapped avocadoes are just perfect when you are on the go. You can grab these bits of health while you are still packing your bag for the office. Or there are times when you are getting ready at 6 pm for a dinner party. You feel hungry but you do not want to overeat before dinner. These bacon wraps come in handy at such rush hours.

SERVES: 2
PREPARATION TIME: 15 min
INGREDIENTS:

Chili powder 1 teaspoon

Brown sugar ¼ cup

Avocado 1

Bacon 4-6 slices

METHOD:

1. Preheat your oven to 425 degrees.
2. Take a medium sized baking dish and line it with foil.
3. Take a small bowl and mix the brown sugar and chili powder.
4. Cut the avocado in half and remove its pit. Cut thin slices of avocado about ¾ inches thick.
5. Cut the slices of bacon into 3-5 pieces.
6. Wrap the bacon slices around the pieces of avocado.
7. Roll the wraps in the mixture of brown sugar and chili.
8. Place the rolls on the baking tray.
9. Cook for 10-15 minutes.
10. Take out the wraps on a plate and stick a toothpick in the center.
11. Serve.

Salmon Baked with Herbs

The herb fragrance while the salmon is baking is sure to get your mouth watering! This makes a lovely light dinner dish. As a bonus, the dish is completed with minimum hassle. If salmon is eaten regularly, it prevents depression and lethargic thinking, and is good for eye health too. Moreover, if you are suffer from insomnia, it will help you have a good sleep. Salmon is called a "happy food" because of the many health benefits it offers.

SERVES: 2
PREPARATION TIME: 30-40 min
INGREDIENTS:
Salmon fillet with skin 12 ounces
Finely chopped shallot 1
Chopped parsley 2 tablespoons
Chopped basil 2 tablespoons
Dried / fresh dill 1 tablespoon
Lemon zest, finely grated 1 tablespoon
Olive oil 1 tablespoon
Sea salt ½ teaspoon
METHOD:

1. An hour prior to your beginning this recipe, you need to do this preparation:
2. Remove salmon from your refrigerator and let it come to room temperature.
3. Take a pan and fill it half with water. Place it on the lower rack of the oven; preheat the oven at a temperature of 250 degrees.

METHOD (to make the herb paste)

1. Chop the parsley, shallot, and basil with other herbs. Mix the lemon zest and olive oil into this mixture.
2. Grease a rack with oil and place it over the baking tray.
3. Position the fillet of salmon on the rack with the skin side facing downwards.
4. Coat the top side of the salmon with a thick layer of the herb mixture. You can coat the sides too if the herb paste does not fall off.
5. Put the salmon in the middle rack of the oven. Bake it for 25-30 minutes.
6. If your fillet is quite thick, it might require more time.
7. Take out the salmon and close the door.
8. Insert a knife in the thickest portion of salmon and check whether it is cooked. If it flakes easily, it is ready. If not, put it back into the oven for further baking. Check again after 5 more minutes.
9. Take out the salmon and cut it into 2-3 pieces. Remove the skin with the help of a spatula.
10. Sprinkle with salt and serve.

Peppermint Bombs

Chocolate and mint are a brilliant combination, and a perfect ending to a lovely meal.

SERVES: 2
PREPARATION TIME: 15-20 min
INGREDIENTS:
Coconut butter ¾ cup
Shredded coconut 1/3 cup
Coconut oil 3 tablespoons
Peppermint extract ½ teaspoon
Cocoa powder 2 tablespoons

METHOD:

1. Combine the coconut butter (melted), shredded coconut, coconut oil (1 tbsp) and peppermint extract.
2. Stir well and pour the mixture into small sweet moulds. Fill the moulds only half way.
3. Place the moulds in the refrigerator for 15 minutes.
4. Mix the coconut oil (2 tbsp) and cocoa powder in a bowl.
5. Take out the moulds from the refrigerator. Pour the cacao mixture into the moulds over the peppermint.
6. Put the moulds back in the refrigerator.
7. When the bombs harden, take them out of the fridge 5 minutes before serving.

Pistachio Almond Fat Bombs

Almonds and pistachios are always a treat. Put them in anything and you can transform even the most boring dish in the world. Your family is bound to love these little morsels. Keep them a secret and surprise your family after dinner. Nobody will be able to resist them.

SERVES: 2
PREPARATION TIME: 15 min
INGREDIENTS:
Cocoa butter ½ cup
Almond butter 1 cup
Coconut butter, creamy 1 cup
Coconut oil 1 cup
Coconut milk, full fat ½ cup
Ghee/ clarified butter ¼ cup
Vanilla extract 1 tablespoon
Salt ¼ teaspoon
Chai spice 2 teaspoons
METHOD:

1. Take a baking dish and line it with parchment paper. Leave a little paper hanging on both sides. It will help you to unmold it easily.
2. Take a saucepan and melt the cocoa butter over low heat.
3. Take a bowl and mix the almond butter, coconut butter, firm oil of coconut, coconut milk, clarified butter, vanilla extract, chai spice, almond extract and salt. Blend the ingredients well.
4. Pour the cocoa butter from the pan into the mixture and combine well.

5. Transfer the mixture into baking dish and spread it evenly.
6. Sprinkle with chopped pistachios (raw).
7. Keep it in the fridge for 4 hours or overnight.
8. Take the pan out next day and cut it into small pieces.
9. Serve chilled.

Mushroom Sauce and Steak

Mushrooms along with steak is just an awesome combination. Try this recipe and you will fall in love with it.

SERVES: 2
PREPARATION TIME: 15 min
INGREDIENTS:
Rib eye steak 2 pounds
Salt 1 teaspoon
Pepper ¼ teaspoon
Butter 1 tablespoon
Port wine 4 ounces
Sliced Mushrooms 10 ounces
Heavy cream 2 ounce

METHOD:

1. Preheat your oven to 450 degrees Fahrenheit.
2. Sprinkle the pepper and salt on both sides of steak.
3. Take a cast iron skillet and heat it on high.
4. Put in butter and let it bubble.
5. Put steak in butter and cook it for 2 minutes on each side.
6. Take out the steak and put it in the oven.
7. Bake the steak in the oven until the desired internal temperature of the steak is reached. It should be 135 degrees for rare.
8. Take the steak out and cover it with a foil.
9. Add port wine to the skillet to deglaze. Scrape off all the tasty bits that are stuck on the skillet.
10. Add mushrooms and heavy cream.
11. Let the sauce simmer and thicken.

12. Pour the sauce over the cooked steak.
13. Serve hot.

Conclusion

After reading so many recipes based on the ketogenic diet, you must be feeling relaxed that you do not have to give up on your favorite foods that contain fat. You can freely eat whatever meat you want. Moreover, there is a wide range of options available for vegans as well. You do not have to give up on your favorite dishes.

The best part of the ketogenic diet is that you can eat meats, cheese, mayonnaise, etc. and just cut down a little on the carbohydrates. The body gradually adapts to utilize fats for energy instead of carbohydrates. It means that you do not have to make any extra effort to shed off the extra fat on your body. Your body will automatically make that effort for you. Carbohydrates make you feel sleepy for hours but fats don't.

When you are on a high carbohydrate diet, the body anticipates high energy sources to keep coming to it. But when you are on a high fat and low carbohydrate diet, your body has to organize itself to mobilize the fats it receives as an energy source.

A very important benefit of this diet is that fats keep you feeling satiated for longer. It means that you eat a lot of fats but actually you do not have to eat all day to satisfy your hunger. But, carbohydrates make you feel hungry again and again. The volume of your food decreases but the amount of calories taken in by your body remains adequate.

Adapting to a ketogenic diet takes at least 2-3 weeks depending upon the person. So please be patient when you start this new lifestyle for yourself.

Ketogenic Miracle

Enhancing Health while Increasing Weight Loss Success

How can you avoid Ketogenic Diet mistakes

By: *Emily Simmons*

Table of Contents

Chapter 1

    What is the Ketogenic Diet?

Chapter 2

    What should you eat?

Chapter 3

    What Can You Expect From the Ketogenic Diet?

Chapter 4

    What, apart from willpower, is needed to start the Ketogenic Diet?
    How to get started

Chapter 5
Chapter 6

    How can you avoid Ketogenic Diet mistakes?

Conclusion

Introduction

Folks, you have this amazing book called *Ketogenic Diet Mistakes You Need to Know* in your hands. You must have already read a lot about the Ketogenic Diet before starting it. Of course, it is always easy to start something, but a lot more difficult to stick to it. This doesn't only apply to difficult things. Many people struggle to see even a small commitment through to the end.

A lot more than determination and willpower are needed to stay committed to the Ketogenic Diet. This book deals with the requirements and hazards of the Ketogenic Diet in full detail. Go through the chapters given in this book. You will not find any dearth of knowledge about this "intimidating" diet. You will hopefully feel more enlightened after reading this book, because it sheds enough light on the concept to chase away all your feelings of intimidation.

Before just jumping into the area that deals with common mistakes, we have given you some general information on the Ketogenic Diet- the foods you should and shouldn't eat, things you must and must not do, and the possible mistakes that you need to learn to watch out for.

It is smarter to learn from the mistakes of others. It saves you much time, energy, and money. Otherwise, when you do not take the precautionary steps and keep making the mistakes, you'll quickly start to feel miserable and will most likely quit the regime.

You have made a smart move by starting with this book. This proves that you are willing to improve your well-being. We have very fast lives these days and it is always better to be prepared beforehand rather than repent later. If you have already started the Ketogenic regime, you still have enough time to learn the hazards in case you have been unintentionally causing trouble for yourself. If you have not yet started it, please take the time to read this Bible of the Ketogenic Diet and only then take your first step. We'll lay any lingering anxieties you may have to rest. Why not invite a few friends along on this health-filled journey and ask them to support you if they are willing? It's always easier to complete the course when you have someone along with you.

Just set aside your inhibitions and let's get started.
Remember to enjoy the journey rather than only look at the target.
Our best wishes are with you!

Chapter 1
What is the Ketogenic Diet?

The Ketogenic Diet, also known as Keto Diet, is based on the concept of eating fewer carbohydrates and more fats. This makes the body produce ketones in the liver that are used as energy. You must be wondering what ketones are. Well, they are the acids or organic compounds which are produced when our bodies start using fats for energy in place of carbohydrates. When our bodies do not have enough glucose obtained from sugar in the blood to transport it into the cells, our bodies use fats instead and break them down to supply us with energy. However, high levels of ketones are harmful for the body, and may lead to a condition called ketoacidosis.

The Ketogenic Diet has been in existence for more than 5 decades, but has risen in popularity in the last few years. It is famously known by many names: Low Carbs Diet, LCHF (Low Carb High Fat Diet), Keto Diet, etc.

When our diets are rich in carbohydrates, our body produces insulin and glucose.

It is easiest for the body to make energy from glucose. Thus, it automatically chooses glucose over any other molecule to convert it into energy. Insulin performs the activity of taking glucose around your body and processes it in your bloodstream. Now, you can understand that since glucose is mainly used as a primary source of energy, fats are not usually used and therefore they are stored in different parts of our bodies. This makes our bodies bulky.

Our normal diet is high in carbohydrates, which provides glucose as the primary source of energy. When we lower the intake of carbohydrates, the body is encouraged to enter into a condition called ketosis. It is a natural process, which is initiated by the body when we consume less food. During this condition, our body produces ketones by breaking down fats taken from the liver.

The primary goal of a well maintained ketogenic diet is to encourage our bodies to enter this state of metabolism. This does not mean that we have to starve for calories, but we do need to cut down on carbohydrates. This has a plus side to it. We can indulge in a lot of fats and still not feel guilty about it. However, we need to look out for some common mistakes, which we will talk about later.

Our bodies are made to be extremely adaptive. We can put them through whatever conditions we have to and they can adjust. Even when we snatch a major portion of carbohydrates from our diet, we will not feel weak once our bodies adapt to the new diet. They will start utilizing ketones as the primary source of energy.

Chapter 2
What should you eat?

If you want to begin the Ketogenic Diet, you will need to plan very well because this diet does not suit everyone. You must have a practicable diet plan before you begin. Whatever you consume depends on how quickly you want to enter into the state of ketosis. The faster you quit carbohydrates, the quicker you will reach ketosis.

Normally, the net amount of carbs specified for the Keto Diet is 20-30 grams every day. You might be wondering, "What are net carbs?" Don't worry. It's really simple. "Net carbs" means the total carbs in your diet minus the amount of fiber. For example, 100 grams of lettuce contains 3 grams of carbohydrates and 1.3 grams of dietary fiber. So, we can deduce that if we subtract 1.3 grams of fiber from 3 grams of carbohydrates, we are left with 1.7 grams of net carbs.

It may be a challenge to stick to a healthy diet low on carbs, particularly when you have just started it. However, owing to the popularity of this diet nowadays, you will not find any shortage of recipes to look for which contain fewer carbohydrates. You can go through the list below of foods friendly to the Keto Diet to help you make the appropriate choices. You must keep one thing in mind: that you have to eat real food, not only food that is low in carbohydrates. Foods like eggs, meats, nuts, vegetables, yoghurt, and some fruits occasionally. Also, you must avoid any kind of processed food which may contain colorings and preservatives.

Following the Ketogenic Diet does not mean that you have to lose weight regardless of the cost. It is all about taking on a healthier lifestyle.

<u>You can eat these things freely:</u>
Wild animals and grass fed animal sources of protein

Grass fed meat simply means that it is the meat of an animal which grazes grass. You can indulge in the grass fed meat of goat, lamb, beef, and venison.

Wild caught seafood and fish, pastured poultry and pork, ghee, gelatin, pastured eggs, and butter. These foods have a high content of omega 3 fatty acids.

You must keep away from farmed fish, meat and sausages covered with breadcrumbs, meat which comes with starchy or sugary sauces, and hot dogs.

You can also eat the offal (heart, liver, kidneys, and meat of other organs) of grass fed animals.

Healthy fats

Saturated fats like tallow, lard, goose fat, duck fat, clarified butter or ghee, coconut oil, butter.

Monounsaturated fat like macadamia, avocado, olive oil.

Polyunsaturated omega 3's, from animal sources like seafood and fatty fish.

Non-starchy vegetables

Cruciferous vegetables like kohlrabi, kale, and radish leaves.

Leafy greens like bok choy, Swiss chard, lettuce, spinach, endive, chives, radicchio, etc.

Celery stalks, cucumber, asparagus, summer squash (spaghetti squash, zucchini), bamboo shoots.

Condiments and beverages

Coffee (with coconut cream or black coffee), still water, black or herbal tea.

Pork rinds for breading.

Mustard, mayonnaise, homemade bone broth, pesto, pickles, homemade fermented foods like kombucha, kimchi, sauerkraut, etc.

All herbs and spices, lime or lemon zest and juice.

Whey protein, egg white protein, grass fed and hormone free gelatin. Keep away from artificial sweeteners, additives, soy lecithin, hormones.

Fruits

Avocado

<u>**You can eat these foods occasionally:**</u>

Fruits, vegetables and mushrooms

Cruciferous vegetables like green and white cabbage, cauliflower, red cabbage, broccoli, fennel, Brussels sprouts, turnips, swede/ rutabaga.

Nightshades (eggplant, peppers, tomatoes).

Root vegetables like parsley root, leek, spring onion, onion, mushrooms, garlic, winter squash like pumpkin.

Sea vegetables like kombu, and nori; okra, bean sprouts, wax beans, sugar snap peas, water chestnuts, globe or French artichokes.

Berries (blueberries, blackberries, strawberries, cranberries, raspberries, mulberries, etc.)

Coconut, rhubarb, olives.

Full-fat dairy and grain-fed animals

Beef, eggs, poultry, and ghee (stay away from farmed pork, as it has high content of omega 6's!)

Dairy products (cottage cheese, full-fat yogurt, sour cream, cream, cheese.)

Stay away from products which are labeled "low-fat". Many of these products are packed with starch and sugar. They do not have any satiating effect.

Bacon. Be cautious of added starches and preservatives. You can consume nitrates if you have antioxidants in your diet.

Seeds and nuts

Macadamia nuts which are low in carbs and high in omega 3's.

Almonds, pecans, walnuts, pine nuts, hazelnuts, flaxseed, sesame seeds, sunflower seeds, hemp seeds, pumpkin seeds.

Brazil nuts (be cautious of their high selenium content, and eat only very small amount of them.

Soy products (fermented)

If you eat any soy products, eat only fermented or non GMO soy products like tempeh, natto, soy sauce or coconut aminos (paleo-friendly).

Green soy beans or edamame, unprocessed black soy beans.

Condiments

Zero carbohydrate healthy sweeteners (Swerve, Stevia, Erythritol, etc.)

Tomato products (sugar free) like passata, puree, ketchup.

Thickeners like xanthan gum, and arrowroot powder. Remember that xanthan gum is not a paleo friendly gum; still it is used by many paleo followers since you need only a small amount of it.

Extra dark chocolate (it is better to take 70% or 90% chocolate, do not take any soy lecithin), carob and cocoa powder.

Do not take mints and chewing gums. Some of them contain carbohydrates.

Some fruits, vegetables, seeds and nuts with limited carbohydrates- depending on your daily limit of carbohydrates

- Root vegetables (carrot, celery root, beetroot, sweet potato, and parsnip)
- Watermelon Cantaloupe / Honeydew melons/ Galia
- Cashew and pistachio nuts, chestnuts
- Very small amounts of dragon fruits, apricots, peaches, apples, nectarines, grapefruits, kiwi berries, kiwifruit, oranges, cherries, plums, figs (fresh), pears

Alcohol

You can drink dry white wine, dry red wine, or unsweetened spirits. However, if you are on a weight loss regime, it is best to avoid them. These drinks should only be taken once you reach the weight maintenance stage.

You must avoid these foods:

It is important to avoid food containing a high content of carbohydrates, processed foods and factory farmed meat.

All kinds of grains and artificial sweets

Avoid whole grains such as wheat, oats, corn, rye, barley, bulgur, sorghum, millet, rice, amaranth, sprouted grains, and buckwheat. This automatically encompasses products made of grains like pasta, pizza, bread, crackers, cookies, etc.

Avoid white potatoes and quinoa

Avoid sugar, sweets, etc. like table sugar, agave syrup, HFCS, ice-creams, sweet puddings, cakes, and sugary soft-drinks

Fish and pork farmed in factories

They have high content of omega 6 fatty acids which causes inflammation in the body. Farmed fish also contains PCBs. You must also avoid fish with a high mercury content.

Artificial sweeteners

Splenda, sweeteners containing Aspartame, Equal, Acesulfame, Saccharin, Sucralose, etc.

Processed foods

Processed foods which contain carrageenan

MSG (it is contained in a few whey protein products

Sulphites in gelatin and dried fruits

BPAs, they are not always labeled

Wheat gluten

Refined oils and fats

Sunflower, safflower, canola, cottonseed, soybean, corn oil, grapeseed

Trans-fats such as margarine

Products labeled low fat, low carbs, zero carbs

Atkins products, diet drinks and soda

Chewing mints and gums may contain a high content of carbs, or they may also contain gluten, artificial additives, etc.

Milk

A very small amount of full fat raw milk is permissible on the Ketogenic Diet.

Other than that, milk is prohibited for many reasons. Among all dairy products, milk is the most difficult one to digest because it contains few good bacteria. (They are destroyed during pasteurization.) Milk may also contain hormones.

Also, milk is high in carbohydrates. There are almost 4-5 grams of carbs in 100 milliliters of milk.

If you want to make tea or coffee, you can put cream in measured amounts.

Though you can drink small quantities of milk, you must make a note of the total carbohydrates.

Sweet drinks and alcohol

Sweet wine, beer, and cocktails must be avoided.

Tropical fruits

Mango, pineapple, papaya, and banana should be avoided.

Fruits high in carbs should also be avoided such as grapes, tangerines, etc.

You must also avoid fruit juices (both packed and fresh). However, you may drink smoothies in limited quantities. Juices are like water with sugar, but smoothies contain fiber, and they are more satiating.

You must also avoid large quantities of dried fruits like raisins and dates. You may consume them in moderate quantities.

Soy products

You must avoid most of the soy products, excluding non-GMO fermented products that are good for health.

Other things to keep away from

You must keep away from wheat gluten which is present in low-carbs foods. You will have to give up bread.

Stay away from cans lined with BPA. If possible, you must look for BPA-free containers like glass jars. BPA is partly responsible for many health ailments like impaired thyroid function, cancer, etc.

[BPA implies bisphenol A. It is a chemical used in industries which make a particular kind of resins and plastics. It is normally found in epoxy resins and polycarbonate plastics. Such plastics are used to make containers that store beverages and food. Epoxy resins are applied on the inside of containers like food cans, water supply lines and bottle tops.

Research has shown that BPA is capable of seeping into beverages and foods from these containers, which is terrible for health. Thus, it is better to avoid products packed in such containers.]

You must avoid other additives like carrageenan, MSG, sulfites.

Chapter 3
What Can You Expect From the Ketogenic Diet?

Benefits of following the Ketogenic Diet:

What benefits do you get from following such a strict diet? There are many. Not only does the Ketogenic Diet help you to lose weight, but it also gives you the following advantages:

Cholesterol: The Ketogenic Diet improves your cholesterol and triglyceride levels, which are mostly linked with the clogging up of arteries.

Weight loss: Since your body burns fat for energy in this diet, your body weight automatically comes down during the state of fasting.

Blood sugar: LDL cholesterol decreases over time with the Keto diet; The symptoms of type 2 diabetes can be controlled over time with the Keto diet

Energy: Fats are more effective and long lasting source molecules to be burned as fuel by our bodies. Since they are a more dependable source of energy, you should feel even more energized on the Ketogenic Diet.

Hunger: Fats keep us satiated for longer hours and we feel hungry less often. Obviously, when we consume less, we gain less weight.

Acne: On a keto diet, you can recognize a drop in skin inflammation and acne lesions in just 12 weeks.

Why physical performance goes down temporarily on a ketogenic diet:

When you begin any new diet, your body needs time to adapt to it. This is also the case with the Ketogenic Diet. When you first start eating food high in fats and low in carbohydrates, you may see some limitations to the physical performance of your body. However, as soon as your body completely adapts to using fats as the main source of energy, you will start to regain your endurance and strength very quickly. Many people are curious about whether they need carbohydrates to build strength and muscles. Absolutely not. When you work out to make muscles, you need to understand how your body processes food to gain mass and strengthen up well. Protein is the key.

Your body storage of glycogen can be refilled when you are on the Ketogenic Diet. This diet allows you to build good muscles, but there is a trick. You have to keep a check on your protein intake. Experts suggest that you must take in between 1.0-1.2 grams of protein for each lean pound of your body mass. You might find it difficult to gain mass on the Ketogenic Diet because the total fat in your body does not increase on the Ketogenic Diet. If for any reason you want to put on weight, you can do it through the Targeted Keto Diet or the Cyclical Keto Diet.

You might encounter some people who argue that performance is affected while you are on a Ketogenic diet. This is not entirely true. There was a study performed on trained cyclists undergoing the Ketogenic Diet. The results showed that their aerobic endurance remained good and was not affected at all. Also, their muscle mass remained the same as it had been when they had started. The cyclists' bodies adapted to the diet through ketosis, and their bodies limited glycogen and glucose storage and utilized fats for converting into energy.

During the time of the research, this group of cyclists was fed on a rigorous diet of proteins, green vegetables, and a good quantity of fats. Thus, even when you do more cardio exercises, the Ketogenic Diet helps you a lot.

The only time when ketosis can make you suffer in performance is when you need give explosive performance. When you need some boost in your workouts, you may take in more carbohydrates by consuming 25-30 grams of the same approximately 30 minutes prior to your training.

Hazards of a ketogenic diet:

You will probably find many people trying to scare you away from a low carbohydrate diet. But don't worry; they're likely under some misconceptions which are more famous than the Keto Diet itself. There have been hundreds of studies conducted with people who have followed the Keto Diet. The studies and research have proved that fewer carbohydrates and more fats are beneficial for health.

Strangely, people confuse the Ketogenic diet with a high carbs and high fats diet- a combination which is dreadful for the body. Obviously, when you eat tremendous amounts of food rich in fats as well as sugars, you are heading towards trouble.

If you have been thinking about going on a low fat diet, please think again. The Ketogenic Diet has been proven to be more effective for losing weight than a low fat diet. If you consume foods rich in carbohydrate content, your body produces glucose naturally. As we have already mentioned, our body finds it easiest to process carbohydrates and therefore, the body will look for them first. This results in immediate storage of excess fat in different parts of the body. This makes you gain weight and also gifts you with other ailments correlated with a high carbs-high fat diet, but not with the Ketogenic Diet.

Just to be safe, please check with a physician if you have any doubts about starting the Ketogenic Diet. You will also need to take precautions if you have a family history of diabetes or kidney ailments, because if you take in more proteins, it will put more strain on the kidneys.

High blood sugar, heart disease and high cholesterol are not the things you need to be concerned about. A high fat, low carbs diet is documented and known for improving blood sugar, cholesterol and reducing heart risks in your body.

What changes does your body undergo during the Ketogenic Diet?

Our bodies are adapted to the simplest routine of processing carbohydrates and utilizing them as energy. As a result, the body has an army of enzymes which are used in this metabolism, while it has only a small amount of enzymes which process fats. Even the enzymes which process the fats, mostly have the job of storing them.

When our bodies suddenly have to adapt to a shortage of glucose and high levels of fats, it is a lot of work for our bodies. They have to build a new army of enzymes adaptive to process fats. However, God has gifted us with amazing bodies which can do wonders when called on to adapt to any situation.

When our bodies are pushed into a state of ketosis, they naturally use what is remaining of the glucose. This implies that our bodies will exhaust up all the glycogen from our muscles, which can temporarily cause weakness or a feeling of low energy. You might feel lethargic for a few days. In the initial few weeks, you may experience mental fogginess, headaches, symptoms of flu (also called Keto-flu), irritability, and dizziness. Some people also called it a PMS for all!

Usually, these sicknesses are a result of your body flushing out electrolytes. Therefore, you may also pass more urine in the initial days of the Ketogenic Diet. You must ensure that you keep up your intake of sodium, and drink plenty of water. You can increase your salt consumption to large amounts. Take salt with everything possible. Doesn't that sound good? You do not have to keep any check on your salt intake. Salt helps your body to retain water and also helps to replenish electrolytes.

The average person who begins the Ketogenic Diet will take approximately 2 weeks to cut down his carbohydrate intake to 25-40 grams. However, it is best if you can cut down the carb intake to as low as 15 grams so that you can get on the right track in just one week. Therefore, the less time you take to reach the state of ketosis, the less time you will have to bear the feeling of sickness.

If you are a regular gym goer, you may notice that you may lose a little endurance and strength at first. As already mentioned, this is normal for everyone. However, you will soon reach sustainable levels of energy throughout the day.

Chapter 4
What, apart from willpower, is needed to start the Ketogenic Diet?
How to get started

When you eat fat rich foods, consume moderate amounts of proteins and few carbs, it has a massive effect on your health. You are already aware of the benefits of the Ketogenic Diet, despite its initial side effects. In the initial weeks, you might crave carbohydrates, but that phase will pass gradually. Artificial sweeteners are linked with sugar cravings. Thus, if you usually consume diet sodas or artificial sweeteners, you will need to flush them out of your system. Having a strong willpower and the right diet chart will help you transform your eating philosophies.

Did you cheat on your diet chart?

Hmm... So, you have finally cheated on your Keto Diet. It's okay once in a while. But ideally, this should not go on forever. If you have been off the track for a few days, you will definitely want to get back to your healthy Keto regime as soon as possible. Obviously, it feels good when you know that you are healthy from the inside.

It sounds simple, but sometimes it can be a monumental challenge. Once you cheat just for a non-Keto meal, you feel dreadful the next morning. You might feel bloated, shaky, and exhausted. Yes, it happens. Remember, when you switched to the Keto Diet, you felt the same sickness. Now when your body has adapted to the Ketogenic Diet, it will definitely shake when it does not get its regular diet of fats. So, now you know that since you have cheated once, you might do it again. Thus, it is better to be prepared for the next time. Take a look at the following tips and note down whichever you find appropriate for you.

1. Whatever you like to do, do not beat yourself up

This is the most important advice given to ketogenic followers. There is a large group of ketogenic disciples who blame themselves for not having enough willpower to manage their new diet. Well, you are a human being and all of us fail sometimes. There is nothing to blame yourself about. We live in a world full of gluten and sugar. We have to face the temptation daily at some place or the other. If you do not give in to these temptations even 80% of times, you are a winner. It is an achievement to have even this much willpower.

Suppose your friend cheated once on their diet. Would you beat them? Never... So why do you do it to yourself? Just keep on trying!

1. Be responsible for your behavior

Do not take the first tip as an excuse. If you ate a bowlful of ice-cream at the party last night, take responsibility for it. If your body feels awful after cheating, positively take responsibility for it. Make a note of situations when you are tempted to cheat. For example, when you leave home for the office, do not forget to take some fat bombs along. If you are tempted to eat due to emotions, or due to boredom, or for some other reason, note down such situations and be prepared for them in advance. Don't allow yourself to become too hungry- when you are already full, you will be less likely to stuff yourself more.

1. Either have a salad for breakfast or do not have breakfast after a night of cheating

After you have cheated on the Keto Diet, you must take a strictly Keto meal after that. If you had a non-Keto meal at night, you might even like to skip your breakfast the next day. Intermittent fasting has been recognized as a healthy practice worldwide. You can eat later when you truly feel hungry. Do not eat just for the sake of eating. Eat when your body demands it. You will not feel weak at all.

Also, eating a plate full of Keto vegetables is just like healing your stomach after you have had an unhealthy meal. But, eat it only if you feel like eating. You will feel rejuvenated.

1. **Make notes**

Remember the good old school days when you used to make notes for every important thing so that you could cram them for exams? Similarly, you just need to note down the good as well as bad feelings you have towards your ketogenic regime. Fix a day in the week to write down your feelings briefly.
If you felt good for several weeks, write it down. If you felt awful after a meal of cheating, then write it down immediately. It is easy to forget your bad feelings once you overcome the inflammation, headaches and stomachaches. This simple practice of writing will give you a much more real and objective picture of your diet.

1. **Go get moving**

When you run or take a brisk walk for a few kilometers to get rid of the hangover after too much to drink, it helps your body break down all the harmful material you dumped into it the previous night. The same process works for food hangovers too. When you have a heavy, unhealthy meal, make sure that you make some time to work out. It does not have to be a vigorous workout, but should at least raise your heart rate a little and work out your bowels. You will definitely feel better once you make this a habit.

1. **Cut down on alcohol**

There is no doubt that alcohol is a toxic substance, even if it is just wine. When you take in alcohol, especially hard drinks, you have a high chance of losing your willpower and cheating on your meals. Thus, it is better to have as little alcohol as you can. Moreover, if you do take it, make sure that you digest it properly and get rid of the hangover.

1. Sip low carb liquids and lots of water frequently

It is advice given regularly by all dieticians, but it needs to be repeated often. We cannot emphasize this fact enough that you can flush out all the unhealthy molecules in your body by drinking appropriate amounts of water. If you are prone to boredom eating and feel like you want to stuff your mouth with something every hour, then you should rather choose warm water or flavored cold water over snacks. Look for your favorite flavors of herbal tea without sweeteners.
If you need something more satisfying, you can try sipping some warm bone broth. This will fill you up without adding any extra carbs to your diet. You can also add some turmeric to the bone broth to add flavor and take advantage of its anti-inflammatory properties.

1. Do not leave home hungry

When you leave home, make sure that you eat something healthy first. When you leave on an empty stomach, you will be more tempted to grab a burger or other fast food. You succumb to your temptations more easily when you are hungry. When you do not feel hungry, you have 90% less chance of cheating on Keto.

1. Do not punish or deprive yourself

Do not go overboard with the Ketogenic Diet and become a maniac. Just because you have started a healthy diet does not mean that you cannot eat when you want to. As already mentioned, if you are prone to boredom eating or emotional eating, keep some healthy substitutes with you. If you feel hungry, then please eat. Eating only a plate of salad a day for weeks at a time is not a good idea at all. These kinds of habits eventually make you even more prone to giving in to your temptations.

1. Find a support group or a buddy

There are many benefits to doing the Keto Diet with friends or with a support group. You get the required emotional support and you become accountable to someone. It is sometimes really difficult to keep promises to yourself. When you make a promise to your conscience, it is much easier to pretend that you never made it and you can just break it anytime. When you declare it to someone else, you feel more strongly that you have to abide by it.

If you cannot find any real friends to support you, you can join any online forum. Such virtual support is also helpful, because obviously real people are there on the other end. You can also get some amazingly easy recipes from these forums.

1. Develop cooking as a hobby

If you have been shying away from cooking throughout your life, now is the right time to pick the hobby up. When you cook something amazing, you feel encouraged to try and cook even more. Motivate yourself and look for some easy and fun recipes to support your Ketogenic Diet.

Chapter 5

What are the common mistakes committed by Keto followers?

As we have already mentioned before, if you have any doubts about the Ketogenic Diet, you must consult your physician. This high fat and low carb diet does not suit everyone. Though you probably know all the benefits of the Ketogenic diet, you also need to know where you can go wrong. Ketones are really beneficial as a fuel for the diaphragm and the heart. The state of ketosis can provide you with great cognitive performance and a good amount of focus. If you are an endurance athlete, this diet can prove extremely beneficial for distance swimming, cycling, ultra-running, or marathons.

However, there are not many resources available around us that can lead us to ketosis without experiencing nutrition deficiency if your Ketogenic diet goes wrong. Moreover, these deficiencies can get really big if you work out a lot. In addition, consuming MCT oil and coconut oil can get really, really boring very soon.

So, you must be thinking, "If there are so many stumbling blocks in my way to reaching the state of ketosis, is this diet worth the effort?" Yes, it is, definitely. It is not as difficult as it sounds. But it is crucial to have a basic understanding of the metabolism of your body and its nutritional needs before your march ahead with this diet plan.

You must also find out about the common mistakes committed by people who are already following this diet. Prepare yourself with a lot of ketogenic recipes and then go ahead and begin your new lifestyle.

Mistake No.1 Being afraid of fat

Obviously you know that you need to consume more fats than ever in the Ketogenic Diet. But the fact is that most of us are not able to overcome the mental block of thinking of fats as evil. The food industry has brainwashed us for many decades that we need to consume as few fats as we can in order to remain healthy. But the fact is that even on a non-Keto diet, we must consume some amount of fats to remain healthy. Even more in the Ketogenic Diet, where we have to derive our energy from fatty acids instead of glucose, we have to consume even more fats without any guilt. Since we are not consuming many carbohydrates, we must not shy away from fats.

Eat full fat cheese, eat the skin of the chicken, soak the broccoli in butter.... yeah... you are right. You have to eat as much fat as you can. The only fats you need to keep away from are vegetable oils like corn and canola. Such oils do not help cure inflammation in our bodies.

Even when you see that you need to consume massive amounts of meat and oils, try to remember that fat is not "evil" for your body. But do consume fats under the right guidance. You would not like to end up getting sick.

Mistake No.2 Consuming an excess of protein

Beginners of the Ketogenic Diet make another common blunder of replacing carbohydrates with proteins. This can lead you to gluconeogenesis, which means that amino acids are converted to glucose. But this is the exact opposite of what we need on a Ketogenic diet. We need to keep the glucose levels at a lower level and speed up the process of making ketones from fatty acids.

The fact is that you actually need to consume very small amounts of protein because fats are protein sparing. That means that our bodies' requirement of protein goes down with the high intake of fats. Thus, you do not need to worry if you are consuming fewer carbs. Do not try to compensate for them with proteins.

Mistake No. 3 Quitting too early

When you enter into the state of ketosis quickly, you might initially suffer from side effects. The changes in metabolism can be really dramatic because every cell of your body has to switch from the metabolism of glucose to fats. Your insulin levels go down due to lower levels of carbohydrates. This also affects your kidneys, which adapt to hold on to the sodium available in the body. When the insulin level is consistently low, the kidneys also shed sodium and water.

This is why it is always recommended that you consume more sodium and drink plenty of water, particularly in the initial phase. It helps to escape the Keto-flu. It is more appropriate if we call the symptoms "symptoms of carbohydrate withdrawal" due to the effect on electrolyte and hormonal balance.

These facts might seem intimidating to you. But you must pledge to yourself that you will not quit regardless of a little sickness in the initial days. You can consume strong bone broth containing high quality salt. You must also take a lot of rest and not work out intensely. Also, drink lots of water rich in minerals.

Moreover, the best advice is that you must go slowly when you begin the Ketogenic Diet. Do not give up when you feel sick during the first couple of weeks, and make sure you get all the recommended blood tests done. This will ensure that your body is not suppressing any health issues that do not appear on the surface.

Mistake No.4 Carbohydrates creep in

It sounds very obvious. But, it is not very simple as it sounds. Carbohydrates can seep in even from those sources which you think are carb-free. If you are fond of buying herbs, spices and vegetables, you might experience an increase in your carbs intake. Some products that you buy from the market with all the best intentions may contain carbs. For instance, factory made salad dressing, tomato sauces, substitutes for milk like almond milk and coconut milk have sugar added in them, meats such as duck meat, starchy vegetables, some kinds of herbal tea- these are just a few products which might contain carbohydrates.

It might become a challenge for you to eat out because many bars and restaurants use dressings, dips and sauces, which have additional sugar or honey. It definitely tastes good but is not good for your diet at all. You must have solid, dependable information for restricting your carbohydrates intake, particularly in the initial phase when your body undergoes drastic changes.

Mistake No.5 Munching processed foods

This mistake is commonly committed by people who have read the Atkins diet (a low carb diet), and observed the foods which are sold online. No doubt that these foods keep your body at low carbohydrate levels and make your life a lot simpler. But the equally true fact is that these foods have high contents of artificial flavors, coloring, sucralose, polydextrose, and many other artificial sweeteners. These things obviously play havoc with your mental and physical health.

You might feel that you are not familiar with half of the ingredients mentioned in the Keto diet list or you are not aware of the shops which supply them. Do yourself a favor and make an effort find them out. The rule of thumb of the Ketogenic Diet is that if you are not able to cook or bake a meal out of these ingredients, then you must keep away from them.

The time is not far away when most of the food companies will start manufacturing foods made out of real ingredients because the trend of being concerned about one's health is reaching its peak really fast. So, be patient and be the pioneer of the Ketogenic Diet among your friends. They should also feel motivated when they see your dedication.

Mistake No.6 Eating the same recipes time and again and panicking when faced with new recipes

In the initial phase, when you feel overwhelmed by eating low carbs foods, you might always want to eat the same "safe" line of foods habitually. This is because you do not have much knowledge and experience of ketogenic recipes. That is why it is always recommended that you prepare yourself with a lot of ketogenic recipes before you start. Suppose you had to eat eggs and bacon for every breakfast and nuts for snacks all the time. Wouldn't you get bored in just a couple of days? This is really common with most Keto practitioners. Even if you are not a Keto follower, you cannot eat the same pizza for breakfast, lunch and dinner over and over again!

Even when you eat low carb foods in your new regime, you must focus on improving your health. This is possible only with a varied and nutritious diet. Every individual is different. If your Keto friend loves bacon for breakfast, you might not like it.

Eat what you love and keep changing your routine. The same routine causes boredom to set in. That's not the only problem, though. Eating the same foods over and over may also cause nutritional deficiencies in your body and you may even become intolerant towards some foods. This would happen especially if you are very stressed or if you are on any kind of medication.

Intolerance for food sets off cramps, bloating, constipation, diarrhea, and many other symptoms. This not only impacts the gut health but also your immune system. The best thing is to keep trying new Keto-friendly foods, even if you have not ever heard of them. For example, chicken liver is a relatively unfamiliar thing for most people. But it's easy to find and to prepare. The long list of Keto-friendly foods can be transformed into many delicious recipes. So don't just stick to a couple of recipes you know. That will make you quit even faster.

Mistake No.7 A lack of planning

One of the major stumbling blocks on the Ketogenic Diet is a lack of planning. If you do not plan well, there is a good chance that you will fail. For example, you are already aware that your kitchen should be well stocked with most of the Keto-friendly ingredients. But what happens when one day you realize that you do not have enough coconut milk in your fridge? You might panic and get frustrated because the shop near the corner street does not sell coconut milk.

Many Keto ingredients which are staples for a low carb diet such as oily fish, olives, coconut oil, ghee, etc. are available only online or in health shops. More supermarkets are coming up with ketogenic products nowadays. Still, you need to plan properly and be well aware that you would need these products. Thus, when you visit the shop next time that stocks Keto goods, you must buy more than you need for just a meal. You can also cook ketogenic recipes in bulk and save on your time as well as money.

Mistake No.8 Getting too obsessed with the diet

Another major obstacle in the Ketogenic diet is being too obsessed with the diet. You might love to plan every last bite of the day in the initial stages. However, this is not practicable. It is feasible though for those patients who have been recommended the Ketogenic Diet due to any medication or sickness like epilepsy. In such ailments, every bite has to be planned without any chance of failure. Otherwise the patient might have to face serious consequences.

However, since you have chosen the Ketogenic Diet yourself, you must not get too stressed over your dietary changes. The new routine should not interfere with your mental balance. Do not become a maniac thinking what your next meal should be or how you can increase your ketones or what you should eat on the vacation next weekend! In order to avoid such craziness, you should sometimes just relax and make a few recipes without counting and weighing. You can also give yourself some more time if you feel so and do not feel guilty about it.

If you remain under mental stress about your food, you will not be able to enjoy the physical benefits of the Ketogenic Diet. Physical benefits take even more time to show up when you have mental turmoil going on.

Mistake No.9 Ignoring the warning signs of your body

People who get obsessed with the changes in their diets can end up measuring ketones and blood glucose in their body and weighing the food every time, making exact plans for meals, etc. They are even literally scared of eating at restaurants where they cannot actually control their food. According to the experts, these people are the ones who mostly ignore the warning signs given by their body.

For example, perhaps you know that there is a particular ketogenic recipe that you do not like and your tummy feels bloated when you eat it. Still, you eat it because you "know" that it is good for your body. As a matter of fact, your body knows better than you do. Do not ignore the signs given by your body. If a food does not make you feel good from inside, then do not eat it.

In another instance, at some stage you might not feel like exerting your body to do high intensity training. If you go ahead just because it was on the chart for the day, you might end up hurting your ligaments.

No meal or training or expert advice can take over your innate intuition and knowledge. Do take the warning signs seriously and do not foolishly stick to your regime even when your body is telling you not to do so.

The Ketogenic Diet or other low carb diets are not suitable for everyone. If you do not feel better than before you switched to the Ketogenic Diet (after the initial phase of sickness, of course) you might like to reconsider your decision.

Mistake No.10 Giving in to social pressure

Our social lives are a big factor which should never underestimate. Even if our friends and family do not mean to pull us back from our healthy regime; they probably will not stop teasing us. We have to listen to comments like, "Oh, come on dear, you are here to party! Don't be a spoil sport. You will not die if you eat just one slice of pizza!" And so we give in.

It is of course impossible to try and explain about the Ketogenic Diet and its benefits every time. Nobody wants to listen to your blabbing and of course, you would also not like to show off your new lifestyle all the time. Although your family knows about the benefits you have experienced from the Ketogenic Diet, they probably still won't stop pushing you to have another piece of cake.

Furthermore, many medical professionals do not understand the true concept of the Ketogenic Diet. However, it is a well-established fact that you can go by the 80/20 rule, and this allows you to have some breaks and enjoy a few treats in moderate amounts. But, when you are completely in ketosis, you will probably find that you truly do not feel like eating anything apart from the stipulated foods. They actually do not make you feel good when you are in ketosis. When you eat a slice of cake during this state, it actually does not feel good.

- **Mistake No.11 Poor timing**

Another crucial factor in determining the success of the Ketogenic Diet is the timing when you start it. You must consider the circumstances that are present when you are about to start this diet. Since the Ketogenic Diet demands a lot of attention, care and rest; you must not start at least a week before something important is expected. For example, if you have a very important meeting in your office next week, do not start it now.

Also, if you are going through a busy season professionally, you must not start this diet. You can begin this regime when you have ample time in hand to rest if you feel frail in the initial phase of keto. When off season times are going on in your profession, then you can think about starting it. This would allow you to take rest or even a holiday if you cannot work at all.

Mistake No.12 Not providing enough time for the body to transition

In the initial week, your bowel habits may change. You may experience constipation or diarrhea, but it will regulate over time. For some people, fiber supplements help in curing stomach problems. But, for others, fiber may not help at all. Thus, you may want to seek personal advice from your physician before eating lots of fiber.

The adaptation may even take up to a month. Many people also experience an energy blast, euphoric feelings, along with a lot of fat loss. Your urine may smell strange and you might also develop some kind of metallic taste in the mouth. However, you do not have to be worried. These changes are a sign that your new diet is working.

Mistake No. 13 Testing ketosis with urine ketone testing sticks

This is a big mistake some people make. Low carbohydrate diet followers have relied on the urine ketone testing sticks for a very long time.

These sticks test the level of acetoacetate your boy is excreting. You may find it extremely thrilling to see the sticks turn dark purple from light pink. It makes you feel good about your body, but unfortunately, these sticks do not show exact results. Moreover, they cannot show the particular type of ketones your body uses as a fuel.

A more accurate test is the blood test for checking beta-hydroxybutyrate. It will give you a better picture of whether you are adapted to keto or not, or if your body is burning ketones and fat for fuel- which is the actual essence of the Ketogenic Diet.

The information you gain about blood ketones rather than urine ketones is absolute gold regarding your performance on your low carbohydrate diet.

Mistake No. 14 Eating too much or too often

It is very common in our society to eat by the clock and to eat much more than it is required to feed our stomachs. You have probably been doing this on your high-carb diet. But it is a blunder if you do the same with your ketogenic diet. When you eat a high fat and low carb diet, your body really does not require food for many hours in a row.

So do not feel worried about it. People often indulge in three full meals in a day along with snacks. Trust the experts' advice, they would never recommend that you eat this much every day.

Your body can eat up the fats it has stored for energy and sustain effectively. You would not feel deprived even if you do not eat. You have to eat food only when you feel hungry.

Mistake No. 15 Falling short of maintaining blood sugar levels

You must be thinking, "Why do I have to measure my blood sugar when I am not a diabetic?" The fact is that every one of us should keep a check on it. When your blood sugar is normalized during ketosis, it keeps your hunger down, regulates your mood and gives you a sense of well-being. Moreover, when your blood sugar is regulated, it is easier to attain nutritional ketosis and vice versa.

Chapter 6
How can you avoid Ketogenic Diet mistakes?

By now, you must have got an idea that you need tons of patience and perseverance to stay healthy with the Ketogenic Diet. Besides this, you also need a few tricks and tips mentioned in the previous chapters to stick to this new lifestyle. It is easy to give in to social pressure and your own temptations, but you have to be determined and convince your friends and family that this is not just a new fad and that you truly want to transform your body for good.

This can happen only when you are yourself convinced that you have chosen the right track. When your family members see the changes in your body and your health, they might also get motivated to adapt this way of eating.

You have already read the common mistakes people commit. To avoid these pitfalls, you must keep the points listed below in mind. Even if you find them repetitive, they have been mentioned to stress the facts you need to remember at all times.

1. Give yourself enough time to adapt

Never ever start the Ketogenic Diet if you do not have enough time to give to your body for adaptation. You must have at least a couple of weeks in hand to overcome the keto fever and other symptoms like constipation and diarrhea. It's probably best not to start this routine just a week before your holiday. It might spoil your holiday mood and make you feel low.
Such things discourage you a lot and get you off the track sooner than ever. You must be motivated enough to keep up with anything new that you pick up.

1. Ask for support from your friends and family

Since you may also experience mood swings due to the drastic changes in your diet, you may want to inform some of your loved ones about your new routine and ask for their cooperation and support.
Your true well-wishers will be more than happy to help you in this important step of your life. You can also ask them to prohibit you from indulging in non-keto food even when you feel tempted to do so.
They may tease you at times, but do not feel disheartened. Be brave and take it in good spirits. When you give cheerful replies to people, they are even happier with you. When you are in a bad mood, alert them of the situation and tell them to beware of you! You would not like to spoil your relationships forever just because of a couple of hours of mood swings. When you take proper precautionary steps without worrying too much, you are bound to succeed.

1. Stay around motivating factors

You must make friends with people who are positive in their lives and do not pull you down all the time. If you stay around negative people, they might turn out to not be your well-wishers. They are not happy to see anyone succeed and will be happy if you fail.

On the other hand, positive people themselves want to succeed in the smallest things in their lives and are happy to see others do so. They encourage you to keep trying even after you fall at times. They will encourage you to rise up and double your efforts. Spend time with both types of people for one week in your life before starting this routine and you will definitely see the difference the two groups make to your outlook.

1. **Keep visiting the physician**

Do not ignore this piece of advice. You might think that you have read enough and gained much knowledge from people around you, but it is always advisable to seek the advice of a physician you trust. It is worth spending the money in advance rather than thinking of saving it. If you end up making any major mistakes in the Ketogenic Diet, you may have to face some serious consequences and pay much more money than you should have.

Also, it is important to visit a trustworthy physician. He must be able to diagnose you properly and give required advice. There are some physicians who deliberately give you the wrong advice so that you fail frequently and visit them more often so that they can make more money. Beware of such doctors.

If you do not have a family physician in your vicinity, ask your friends who have been following the Ketogenic Diet lately. By all means, get help from internet forums, but please also follow the advice of your doctor.

1. **Do not go maniac**

Yes, you have taken a major step in your life, but nobody would like to see you going nuts over this new ketogenic diet. This fact cannot be stressed enough that we advocate this diet only to see you healthier, and not to see you getting obsessed with ketones and ketosis. You need to make peace with your eating habits. If you do not feel motivated enough to follow this regime, think again if you really want to do it for the rest of your life.

Your body must feel good after making so much effort. If this is not the case, you must seek the advice of your friends and family who have the know-how of the Ketogenic Diet. They might enlighten you if you are not able to decide. But do give yourself ample time to adjust before you want to re-think.

It is always easy to step back once you have decided to do something, but it is not so easy to get back to the same milestone once you have crossed it.

1. Keep yourself well equipped

As you must have already read, keep your kitchen well stocked in advance so that you do not fall short of supplies when you need to cook anything. Since this diet is almost entirely based on fats, it might prove a little expensive for you. Thus, it is better to buy things in larger quantities to save money. Groceries always prove cheaper when bought in bigger packets and of course, they last much longer.

Find stores online which keep groceries specifically for the Ketogenic Diet. You'll probably get your stuff from such stores at much cheaper rates than you would at the local supermarket. Such stores cater to the needs of the Ketogenic Diet followers and stock products required by them. They also procure the groceries at cheaper prices and hence supply them to you at comparatively competitive rates. An occasional supplier of ketogenic supplies will charge much higher than the things are worth. Hence, make an effort and find out places that suit you and your budget.

When you keep the pitfalls and precautionary measures in mind, you will be less likely to fail. It is always better to be well prepared rather than repent later. Keep on the right track and you will definitely reap the fruits soon.

Conclusion

After reading this entire book on the Ketogenic Diet: *Ketogenic Diet Mistakes You Need to Know*, you must be feeling more at ease. It is always good to hear from a reliable source about an important thing that you have been anxious about. The Ketogenic Diet is not at all mysterious in itself but people who have not succeeded in it, have made it so. They have spread such myths about the Ketogenic Diet that even those who have the guts to start it, have to think twice before doing it.

All of us have at least enough willpower to take any new step. The rest of the journey is covered with the help of new milestones and support from our family and friends. You do not need to panic about this diet. Every single human being among us is capable of achieving much more they can imagine. Even the biggest deeds of the world were started as baby steps towards achieving something new. Perseverance and good intentions lead people to achieve what they have always wanted.

Have you ever read the autobiography of an athlete or an Olympic winner? Most of them come from humble backgrounds. They just have big dreams. In the initial stages of their career, even they are doubtful about their success, but as the time passes and they stay patient and keep up the hard work, all their efforts pay off well. Similarly, even if you are an ordinary person with no Olympic aspirations, you cannot underestimate your determination and your motivation. All of us want to have a healthy body and remain disease free throughout our lives. But only a few of us are able to achieve it. It's not that those who have been successful in achieving the state of ketosis have not faced any obstacles. It is just a matter of facing these troubles bravely and overcoming your temptations. The victorious keto-followers have resisted their temptations well. Eventually, when you are able to say, "No, thank you" to mouthwatering cuisines for quite some time, you even start disliking that type of food.

Thus, just keep your eyes on the end results that you are going to have a good body once you have your ketones working for you instead of carbohydrates. I'm sure you will be able to make an effort with even more dedication than you think. Good luck with this life transforming ketogenic diet!

The Ketogenic Mediterranean Diet
Healthy and Delicious Ketogenic Mediterranean
Diet Recipes For Extreme Weight Loss

Disclaimer:

The information presented in this book represents the views of the publisher as of the date of publication. The publisher reserves the rights to alter update their opinions based on new conditions. This report is for informational purposes only. The author and the publisher do not accept any responsibilities for any liabilities resulting from the use of this information. While every attempt has been made to verify the information provided here, the author and the publisher cannot assume any responsibility for errors, inaccuracies or omissions. Any similarities with people or facts are unintentional.

Table of Contents
The Ketogenic Mediterranean Diet
Healthy and Delicious Ketogenic Mediterranean Diet Recipes For Extreme Weight Loss
Table of Contents
Introduction
Chapter 1
The Ketogenic Mediterranean Diet
Chapter 2
Ketogenic Mediterranean Breakfast Recipes
Mediterranean Breakfast with Mushrooms and Tomato
Red Pepper and Goat Cheese Frittata
Breakfast Pizza Skillet
Cauliflower Crust Stromboli
Jalapeño and Cheddar Cauliflower Muffins
Mediterranean Breakfast with Peaches, Ricotta and Honey
Ingredients:
Directions:
Swiss Chard Omelet
Ingredients:
Directions:
Egg-Crust Vegetarian Breakfast Pizza
Spinach, Ham and Egg Whites Frittata Recipe
Tasty Breakfast Casserole with Tomatoes, Green Pepper and Feta Cheese
Healthy Breakfast with Spinach and Cheese
Chapter 3
Ketogenic Mediterranean Lunch Recipes
Italian Roasted Sausage with Vegetables
Halibut with Lemon-Fennel Salad
Mediterranean Shrimp with Charred Tomato Relish
Italian Chicken Soup

Garlic Parmesan Zucchini and Tomato Bake
Greek Salad
Mediterranean Salmon
Baked salmon topped with healthy vegetables tastes fantastic. Check out this preparation method and see that it is as good as promised.
Preparation time: 5 minutes
Cooking time: 22 minutes
Serves: 4
Low Carb Tasty Stuffed Bell Peppers
Ingredients:
Spinach Salad with Chicken, Avocado and Goat Cheese
Ingredients:
Spinach Stuffed Chicken Breasts
Directions:
Portobello Mushrooms with Mediterranean Stuffing
I am sure these stuffed mushrooms will quickly become a favorite. Hot, warm or cool, they are
Roasted Vegetables with Lamb
Chapter 4
Ketogenic Mediterranean Dinner Recipes
Mediterranean Low-carb "Risotto"
Mediterranean Tilapia with Olive and Almond Tapenade
Salmon with a Warm Tomato-Olive Salad
Pork Tenderloin with Olive-Mustard Tapenade
Italian Sausage, Peppers and Onions
Directions
Grilled Pesto Shrimp Skewers
Grilled Chicken with Tomato Mixture
Zucchini, Tomato and Mozzarella Pie
Baked Cod with Roasted Vegetables
Mediterranean Chicken and Vegetable Kebabs

Directions:
Seared Mediterranean Tuna Steaks
Beef Tenderloin with Mustard and Herbs
Ingredients:
Directions:
Chapter 5
Ketogenic Mediterranean Snack Recipes
Low Carb Cabbage Patties
Low Carb Turkey Patties
Ingredients:
Directions:
Zucchini Parmesan Crisps
Ingredients:
Directions:
Tuna and Zucchini Patties
Roasted Broccoli and Tomatoes
Preparation time: 5 minutes
Cooking time: 12 minutes
Serves: 4
Ingredients:
Directions:
Mediterranean Canapés with Cranberries and Goat Cheese
Tomato-Basil Skewers
Conclusion

KETOGENIC DIET 3 BOOKS IN 1 THE COMPLETE HEALTHY AND DELICIOUS RECIPES COOKBOOK BOX SET

Introduction

I want to thank you and congratulate you on downloading this book: "The Ketogenic Mediterranean Diet".

Many people think that losing weight is all about diets and food. However, people are often exhausted and disappointed by the diet they are following. This is mainly due to the fact that most diets are "fake", and many hit hard on your pockets! With this cookbook we aim to break all stereotypes about dieting and weight loss.

In this book you will find some wonderful recipes incorporating healthy and nutritious food that you can start your dietary intake with. As you will notice, we have put the emphasis on fish, poultry and beef (enabling you to maintain a good intake of protein), and also on fresh vegetables, such as spinach, carrots, cucumbers, cabbage, broccoli etc. We will also present to you some of the healthiest and easiest preparation methods in cooking, thus ensuring that you will make your food both tasty and fulfilling.

This cookbook offers you a wide range of recipes that can be served as a solid breakfast and a hearty lunch, some that will go well as a dinner treat or a light supper. The following chapter will briefly describe to you the concept of The Ketogenic Mediterranean Diet, and it will convince you to not only change your meal plan, but also your lifestyle.

Chapter 1
The Ketogenic Mediterranean Diet

The Ketogenic Mediterranean Diet is more than just a diet, it is a lifestyle change. But for some, it has been their way of life since they were born. People living in the Mediterranean region have had this unique diet for thousands of years. It consists of foods like fruits, vegetables, fish, olive oil, whole grains and red wine. In addition, combining The Ketogenic Diet with the Mediterranean diet is more than just a fat-burning machine, it is one of the healthiest ways to eat. Firstly, let's explore what The Ketogenic Diet is.

The Ketogenic Diet mainly reduces carbohydrates for the body to enter a stage known as ketosis. At this stage, the body naturally burns fat without leaving the individual feeling starved. Because the body is getting all the nutrients it needs to survive, it is happy and thus does not enter into starvation mode. After the initial first stage of The Ketogenic Diet, carbohydrates can gradually be added back in, but the weight should stay off.

Secondly, what is ketosis? It is a harmless state within the body that is completely natural and used to occur when food sources were not as plentiful. Ketosis is a state in which the body uses the stored fat rather than carbohydrates for energy because the carbohydrates are missing from the body. Once the fat is metabolized into fuel, compounds known as ketones form; some of these are used as a glucose substitute, and others are flushed out of the body naturally.

Thirdly, why should you put yourself through the cutting out of carbs and practicing The Ketogenic Mediterranean Diet? The diet is simple to follow and has unlimited amounts of high-protein and fatty foods. Statistically, people have less trouble with hunger on this diet and there is better weight loss results short-term compared to other diets. People with diabetes report lower blood glucose levels and lower blood pressure. Even people who experience hyperinsulinemia (high insulin levels) report that they benefit from this diet. Levels of HDL, or good cholesterol, increase while bad cholesterol decreases, and more people are likely to stick with this diet than any other diet. Finally, people who follow The Ketogenic Mediterranean Diet are less likely to return to unhealthy eating after they've tried this lifestyle.

Those are some pretty enticing reasons to try this diet out. What's more enticing are the foods that you're allowed to eat. The following is a list of foods, separated by food groups, which people on the Ketogenic Mediterranean Diet can enjoy.

Protein (Unlimited Amounts)

Protein is able to be consumed in unlimited amounts because it does not have any of the detrimental carbohydrates, and it keeps the body healthy. Avoid protein products that have been processed and only eat until you feel satisfied, not stuffed full!

- Beef
- Chicken
- Fish
- Eggs
- Seafood
- Pork
- Turkey

Vegetables

When choosing vegetables for The Ketogenic Mediterranean Diet, try to choose ones that would commonly go in a salad or are cooked alone. Always make sure to weigh vegetables before they are cooked in order to get the full nutritional information. It is recommended that you stay away from canned vegetables as they have added sodium and preservatives.

- Salad Vegetables
    - Radishes
    - Mushrooms

- Lettuce
- Spinach
- Tomatoes
- Cucumbers
- Parsley
- Celery
- Scallions
- Arugula
- Chard
- Endive
- Avocados
- Sweet pepper
- Olives
- Radicchio
- Carrots
- Cooking Vegetables
  - Summer Squash
  - Broccoli
  - Onions
  - Tomatoes
  - Cauliflower
  - Eggplant
  - Asparagus
  - Brussels Sprouts

Fish

Fish should make up half the amount of your daily protein intake in the diet, and it is better to eat fresh fish. However, canned fish is still acceptable as long as it is not high in sodium. Some of the more beneficial fish available that have higher omega-3 fatty acids are:

- Sardines
- Trout

- Salmon
- Herring
- White Tuna/Albacore
- Swordfish
- Sea Bass
- Halibut
- Mackerel

Nuts and Seeds

These should be used as a garnish or as a snack.

- Pecans
- Almonds
- Walnuts
- Macadamia Nuts
- Brazil Nuts
- Hazelnuts
- Spanish Peanuts
- Peanuts
- Pine Nuts
- Pistachios
- Pumpkin Seeds in Shell
- Sunflower Seeds

Wine

Wine is a big part of the Mediterranean Diet; however, it should not be abused. Drinking a glass of red wine at night is the most that should be consumed daily. If you are unable to consume wine, there are some acceptable alternatives listed below the wine list. Some red wines are better than others, such as:

- Wine
    - Burgundy

- Cabernet Sauvignon
- Merlot

Cheese

Do not choose non-fat or low-fat cheese. Cheese should be whole milk and regular. Some acceptable cheeses are:

- Swiss
- Mozzarella
- Provolone
- Monterey
- Cheddar
- Blue
- Parmesan
- Colby
- Brie
- Gouda
- Parmesan
- Feta
- Cottage
- Ricotta

Additional Foods

Spices, condiments and other daily foods available in The Ketogenic Mediterranean Diet that can be consumed in an unlimited amount include:

- Pepper
- Genuine Mayonnaise
- Vinegar (Cider, Red Wine, Or Distilled)
- Balsamic Vinegar
- Butter
- Plant Oils (Strongly Favor Olive Oil)

- Yellow Mustard
- Salad Dressing
- Salt
- Worcestershire Sauce
- A.1. Steak Sauce
- Paprika
- Cinnamon
- Ginger
- Cilantro
- Anise
- Spanish Saffron
- Lemon Or Lime Juice
- Turmeric
- Mint
- Garlic (3 Cloves Daily)
- Dill Pepper
- Cumin
- Parsley
- Sumac

Some key points to remember with The Ketogenic Mediterranean Diet are:

✓ Do not eat just the same couple of things (variety is key);

✓ Do not use anything that is low-fat, you can continue drinking coffee or tea (but use high fat cream or half-and-half);

✓ Remember that you will be eating a lot of salads.

While The Ketogenic Mediterranean Diet is safe, remember to keep listening to your body and adjust your meals within the diet if you are feeling overly starved or overly full. Keep in mind that you are doing this for a healthier you, which is right around the corner with The Ketogenic Mediterranean Diet!

Chapter 2
Ketogenic Mediterranean Breakfast Recipes
Mediterranean Breakfast with Mushrooms and Tomato

Reading the list of ingredients you can understand that you are about to make an absolutely delicious breakfast, which is full of vitamins and proteins.

Preparation time: 5 minutes
Cooking time: 15 minutes
Serves: 1
Ingredients:
½ cup egg whites
3 tablespoons olive oil
½ cup thinly sliced mushrooms
½ medium tomato, thinly sliced
Salt and pepper, to taste
½ cup crumbled fresh goat cheese, or cheese of your choice
Directions:

1. Preheat the oven to 400°F (200°C).
2. Add the egg whites to a small bowl, season with salt and pepper, and beat until soft peaks have formed.
3. Add the olive oil to a large oven proof pan and set over a medium-high heat. Stir in the mushrooms and cook until tender, about 5 minutes.
4. Top the mushrooms with tomato slices.
5. Add the crumbled cheese into the egg mixture, slightly stir, and pour evenly over the tomatoes.
6. Transfer the pan to the preheated oven and bake for 7-8 minutes.
7. Remove the pan from the oven and carefully flip the dish over onto a serving plate.

Red Pepper and Goat Cheese Frittata

Frittata is an essential part of the Mediterranean breakfast. It is quick and easy to prepare, and very healthy.

Preparation time: 5 minutes
Cooking time: 8 minutes
Serves: 4
Ingredients:
1 bunch scallions, trimmed and sliced
2 cloves garlic, minced
6 eggs, beaten
½ cup goat cheese, crumbled
1 cup red bell pepper, sliced
2 tablespoons fresh basil, finely chopped
½ teaspoon salt
¼ teaspoon black pepper
Directions:

1. Preheat the broiler.
2. Add the eggs, garlic and basil to a medium bowl, season with salt and pepper and mix to combine.
3. Coat a large ovenproof skillet with cooking spray.
4. Add the bell pepper and green onions and sauté over a medium heat until the green onions are lightly wilted, for 1-2 minutes.
5. Pour the egg mixture over the vegetables and cook for a couple of minutes, without stirring.
6. Gently lift the edges of the frittata to allow any uncooked egg to pour underneath.
7. Once the bottom of the frittata is lightly brown, sprinkle the top of the frittata with cheese. Place the pan in the oven and

grill for about 3 minutes.
8. When it is lightly golden, remove and let the dish stand for 10 minutes before serving.

Breakfast Pizza Skillet

This is a simple, quick and very delicious recipe that offers a great mix of ingredients. It is an ideal breakfast for a weekend morning.

Preparation time: 5 minutes
Cooking time: 20 minutes
Serves: 6
Ingredients:
1 lb (454g) bulk Italian sausage
1 medium tomato, thinly sliced
½ cup mushrooms, sliced
½ cup onion, chopped
½ cup green pepper, chopped
½ teaspoon salt
4 eggs
Pepper to taste
1 cup cheddar cheese, shredded

Directions:

1. In a large frying pan, roast the sausage over a medium-high heat until golden brown on all sides.
2. Add the green pepper and onion, season with salt and pepper, and let it cook over a medium heat for about 5 minutes.
3. Add the mushrooms and stir to combine.
4. In a small bowl, beat the eggs and pour over the fried sausage mixture.
5. Top the mixture with tomato slices and shredded cheese. Place the lid on the pan and cook over a medium heat for about 10 minutes.

Cauliflower Crust Stromboli

This healthy and tasty dish with cauliflower and mozzarella cheese can be served as a complete breakfast or as a side dish to any meal.

Preparation time: 10 minutes
Cooking time: 30 minutes
Serves: 4
Ingredients:
Cauliflower crust
1 small head cauliflower, cut into small florets
1 free-range organic egg, lightly beaten
½ cup (1.7oz/50g) shredded mozzarella cheese
½ teaspoon fine grain sea salt
½ teaspoon dried oregano
¼ teaspoon ground black pepper
Filling
3 tablespoons tomato sauce
½ cup mozzarella cheese
7-8 slices ham
Grated Parmesan cheese
Dried Oregano (to garnish)
Directions

1. Preheat oven to 450°F (220°C) and position a rack in the middle of the oven.
2. Line a baking dish with parchment and coat it with olive oil. Set aside.
3. Place the cauliflower florets in a blender and pulse until they look like rice.
4. Place the ground cauliflower in a microwave-safe dish and microwave for 7 minutes on high, until crisp-tender.
5. Transfer the cauliflower rice onto a working surface lined with a tea towel and press to squeeze out as much liquid as you can.

6. Place the drained cauliflower rice in a medium bowl. Add the mozzarella and egg, and season with the oregano, salt and pepper. Stir until the ingredients are well combined.
7. Place the cauliflower mixture into the prepared baking dish and spread to form a large rectangle.
8. Bake in the preheated oven for 10 minutes.
9. Remove the baking dish from the oven and top the crust with tomato sauce. Ensure you leave a 2-inch border on one side.
10. Sprinkle the dish with half of the grated mozzarella, followed by the ham, and then spread the remaining mozzarella over the dish.
11. Using a plastic spatula, lift the cauliflower crust from one side and fold into a Stromboli.
12. Make sure the Stromboli is in the dish seam side down.
13. Sprinkle the Stromboli with some oregano and Parmesan cheese and bake in the oven for another 10 minutes.
14. Let it stand for at least 10 minutes, then slice and serve warm.

Jalapeño and Cheddar Cauliflower Muffins

Your kids will adore these healthy cauliflower muffins, full of vitamins and nutrients. They are just as good on the second day as they are straight from the oven.

Preparation time: 50 minutes
Cooking time: 30 minutes
Makes: 12 muffins
Ingredients:
2 cups raw cauliflower, finely blended
2 tablespoons minced jalapeño
2 eggs, beaten
2 tablespoons olive oil
⅓ cup grated parmesan cheese
1 cup grated mozzarella cheese
1 cup grated cheddar cheese
1 tablespoon dried onion flakes
¼ teaspoon salt
¼ teaspoon black pepper
½ teaspoon garlic powder
½ teaspoon baking powder
¼ cup coconut flour

Directions:

1. Preheat the oven to 375°F (180°C).
2. Coat 12 muffin cups with oil.
3. In a large bowl, mix together the jalapeño, cauliflower, eggs and olive oil.
4. Stir in the grated cheeses.
5. Add the onion flakes, baking powder, garlic powder, coconut flour, salt and pepper, and mix until blended.
6. Spoon the mixture evenly into the prepared muffin cups and bake in the oven until the tops of muffins are golden brown, for approximately 30 minutes.
7. Turn off the oven but don't remove the muffin pan. Let it sit for 30-40 minutes to firm up.
8. Serve the muffins warm or cold.

Mediterranean Breakfast with Peaches, Ricotta and Honey

Fried peaches with nuts, ricotta and honey is a great way to start your day, or to finish a delicious meal.

Preparation time: 2-3 minutes
Cooking time: 5 minutes
Serves: 1

- **Ingredients:**

1 large or 2 small peaches or nectarines per person
Ricotta (crumbly sort best)
1 teaspoon honey
½ tablespoon pistachios or almonds, chopped
Fresh thyme sprig

- **Directions:**

1. Halve the washed peaches and gently pit them.
2. In a griddle, fry the peaches until they are crisp and tender.
3. Transfer onto a serving plate. Top with a dollop of ricotta, drizzle with the honey and garnish with chopped nuts and the fresh thyme sprig.

Swiss Chard Omelet

This hearty and flavorful omelet can easily be made in 25 minutes and will satisfy everyone.

Preparation time: 10 minutes
Cooking time: 15 minutes
Serves: 4 to 6
Ingredients:
6 tablespoons olive oil
1 yellow onion, finely chopped
1 lb Swiss chard, stems removed and leaves coarsely shredded
7 eggs
1 cup grated Parmigiano-Reggiano cheese
1 garlic clove, finely chopped
2 tablespoons fresh flat-leaf parsley, chopped
Salt, to taste
Freshly ground pepper, to taste
8 to 10 small black olives

Directions:

1. Add 3 tablespoons of the olive oil to a large skillet and set over a moderate heat.
2. Add the onion and cook until tender, 2 minutes.
3. Stir in the Swiss chard and cook until wilted.
4. Reduce the heat to low and cook for about 5 minutes, stirring frequently. Remove from the heat and let the dish cool.
5. In a medium bowl, beat the eggs until frothy. Mix in the parsley, garlic and half of the cheese. Season with salt and pepper.
6. Add the chard mixture and mix to coat.
7. Rinse the skillet, dry with a kitchen towel and place over a low heat. Add the remaining olive oil.
8. When the oil begins to shimmer, stir in the egg mixture.
9. Let this cook for about 4 minutes until the omelet has set at the edges.
10. Gently flip the omelet to cook on the other side. Add the remaining cheese by spreading it evenly over the top of the omelet and cook until melted, for about 3 minutes.
11. Transfer the omelet onto a serving plate. Garnish with the black olives, slice and serve hot.

Egg-Crust Vegetarian Breakfast Pizza

A very interesting and rich combination of mushrooms, black olives and mozzarella cheese. Enjoy!

Preparation time: 15 minutes
Cooking time: 17 minutes
Serves: 2
Ingredients:
4oz (120g) Crimini mushrooms, sliced
3 teaspoons olive oil
6 black olives, sliced
¼ green bell pepper, thinly sliced
1oz (30g) Mozzarella
2 eggs, beaten
Spike Seasoning, to taste (about ½ teaspoon)
¼ teaspoon dried oregano, to taste

Directions:

1. Preheat the broiler.
2. Rinse the mushrooms, drain and cut into slices.
3. Add 2 teaspoons of the olive oil to a large skillet and set over a medium-high heat.
4. Add the mushrooms and cook until golden and crisp-tender, for about 7 minutes. Remove the mushrooms to a cutting board
5. In a small bowl lightly beat the eggs. While the mushrooms cook slice the olives and the bell pepper, and cut the mozzarella into chunks.
6. Add the remaining olive oil to the skillet and set over a medium-high heat.
7. Add the beaten eggs, season with the oregano and Spike seasoning, and cook for 2-3 minutes.
8. Add half the green peppers, half of the mushrooms, half of the olives and half of the cheese.
9. Repeat the process.
10. Place the lid on the skillet and cook until the cheese is melted and the eggs are cooked, for about 4 minutes.
11. Transfer the pan to the oven and broil until the cheese has melted and the top of the frittata is golden-brown, for about 2-3 minutes.
12. Transfer to a plate and serve hot.

Spinach, Ham and Egg Whites Frittata Recipe

If you are on the Ketogenic diet and still thinking of what to make for breakfast, this great frittata recipe is the one for you!

Preparation time: 5 minutes
Cooking time: 25 minutes
Serves: 6
Ingredients:

2 cups egg whites
½ cup lean ham, diced
1 5oz bag fresh baby spinach, washed and chopped
¾ cup reduced fat smoked Gouda cheese, shredded
2 leeks, white and light green parts only, diced
2 teaspoons fresh dill, finely chopped
1 teaspoon garlic powder
1 teaspoon fresh lemon zest
½ teaspoon salt
¼ teaspoon freshly ground pepper

Directions:

1. Set the oven rack in the upper third of oven and preheat to 450°F (230°C).
2. In a medium bowl, beat the egg whites, garlic powder, salt and pepper.
3. Coat a large ovenproof skillet with cooking spray.
4. Add the fresh dill, leeks and lemon zest and sauté, stirring constantly, until tender, for about 3-4 minutes.
5. Add the ham and spinach and cook for a minute.
6. Once the spinach is wilted, pour the egg mixture over the sautéed vegetables. While cooking, lift the edges of the frittata so the uncooked egg can flow underneath.
7. Top the frittata with the cheese, place in the oven and bake for 10 minutes.

8. Remove from the oven and let the frittata stand for 5 minutes before serving.

Tasty Breakfast Casserole with Tomatoes, Green Pepper and Feta Cheese

This marvelous breakfast recipe combines tomatoes, green pepper and crumbled Feta cheese on top.

Preparation time: 10 minutes
Cooking time: 45 minutes
Serves: 4-6
Ingredients:
1 green bell pepper, seeded and cut into thin strips
Olive oil, for brushing the baking pan
½ teaspoon dried oregano
1 cup cherry tomatoes, halved
¾ cup Feta cheese, crumbled
10 eggs
Salt and freshly ground black pepper for seasoning the eggs
Directions:

1. Preheat oven to 375°F (190°C).
2. Coat a round baking pan, including the sides, with olive oil.
3. Place the green pepper in the baking pan, sprinkle with the dried oregano and roast in the oven for 7-8 minutes.
4. In a small bowl, beat the eggs until frothy. Season with salt and black pepper.
5. Add the cherry tomatoes to the baking dish, slightly mix with the green pepper and roast in the oven for another 12-15 minutes, until the tomatoes have shriveled.
6. Top the roasted vegetables with the crumbled Feta cheese and then add the beaten eggs.
7. Place the pan back in the oven and bake for about 25 minutes, until the eggs are set and the top is golden brown.
8. Remove from the oven, slice and serve warm.

Healthy Breakfast with Spinach and Cheese

This is a delicious recipe for a Sunday brunch. The spinach and onions marry the Muenster cheese in the best possible way in this dish.

Preparation time: 20 minutes
Cooking time: 30 minutes
Serves: 4
Ingredients:
1 tablespoon olive oil
1 onion, chopped
5 eggs, beaten
1 (10oz) package frozen chopped spinach, thawed and drained
3 cups Muenster cheese, shredded
¼ teaspoon salt
⅛ teaspoon ground black pepper

Directions:

1. Preheat oven to 350ºF (175ºC).
2. Gently coat a 9 inch baking dish with oil.
3. Add the olive oil to a large frying pan and set over a medium-high heat.
4. Stir in the onions and sauté for a few minutes, stirring occasionally.
5. Add the spinach and sauté until the onions are tender.
6. Whisk together the eggs with the cheese and season with the salt and pepper. Add the spinach mixture and mix to coat.
7. Pour the mixture into the prepared baking dish and bake in the oven until the eggs are set, 25-30 minutes.
8. Let the dish cool for 10 minutes before slicing and serving.

Chapter 3
Ketogenic Mediterranean Lunch Recipes

Italian Roasted Sausage with Vegetables

Enjoy Italian sausage flavored with Mediterranean spices. Garlic, paprika, parsley, rosemary and, turmeric, red and yellow peppers green onion promise an interesting experience.

Preparation time: 5 minutes
Cooking time: 7 minutes
Serves: 4
Ingredients:
8oz (230g) Italian sausage
1 small onion, thinly sliced
6 tablespoons olive oil
1 small red bell pepper, diced
1 small yellow bell pepper, diced
Salt and ground black pepper, to season
3 cloves garlic, pasted
1 teaspoon paprika
1 tablespoon rosemary, finely chopped
2 tablespoons flat-leaf parsley, finely chopped

Directions:

1. Add 3 tablespoons of the olive oil to a large shallow roasting pan and set over a medium-high heat.
2. Add the onions and garlic and sauté until light golden and tender, 2 to 3 minutes. Add the peppers and cook for another 2 minutes.
3. Stir in the sausage and paprika, and season with the salt and pepper. Cook for about 2 minutes whilst stirring frequently.
4. Add the rosemary and then, using a spoon, press the mixture into the pan to brown the bottom, and then stir to divide the crispy bits.

5. Sprinkle the mixture with the chopped parsley.
6. Transfer to a serving dish and drizzle with the remaining olive oil.
7. This dish is great to serve hot or at room temperature.

Halibut with Lemon-Fennel Salad

This delicious fish dish is perfect for any family gatherings. The lemon fennel salad provides an interesting and refreshing taste to this dish.

Preparation time: 10 minutes
Cooking time: 10 minutes
Serves: 4
Ingredients:
1 teaspoon ground cilantro
½ teaspoon salt
½ teaspoon ground cumin
¼ teaspoon freshly ground black pepper
5 teaspoons extra-virgin olive oil
2 garlic cloves, minced
4 (6oz) halibut fillets
2 cups thinly sliced fennel bulb (about 1 medium bulb)
¼ cup thinly sliced red onion (vertically sliced)
2 tablespoons fresh lemon juice
1 tablespoon chopped flat-leaf parsley
1 teaspoon fresh thyme leaves

Directions:

1. In a small bowl, mix together the cilantro, salt, cumin and black pepper.
2. In a separate small bowl, combine the garlic and 2 teaspoons of olive oil. Mix in 1½ teaspoons of the spice mixture made in step 1.
3. Coat the halibut fillets with this spice mixture.
4. Add 1 teaspoon of oil to a large frying pan and set over a medium-high heat.
5. When it begins to shimmer, place the fish in the pan and fry for 5 minutes per side.

6. Mix together the fennel, the remaining oil, the remaining spice mixture, the lemon juice, parsley, onion and thyme leaves in a medium salad bowl.
7. Place the fish on a serving plate, add the salad and enjoy.

Mediterranean Shrimp with Charred Tomato Relish

Grilled shrimp with green tomatoes, plum tomatoes and jalapeño pepper can be served as a healthy and delicious lunch or dinner.

Preparation time: 40 minutes
Cooking time: 15 minutes
Serves: 4
Ingredients:
2 garlic cloves, minced
4 ripe plum tomatoes, halved
2 medium green tomatoes, halved
3 tablespoons vegetable oil
20 extra-large shrimp, peeled, deveined, tails left on
2 tablespoon fresh lime juice
1½ tablespoons ginger, peeled and grated
1 tablespoon fresh jalapeño pepper, minced
1 tablespoon basil, chopped
Coarse salt
1 tablespoon cilantro, chopped
Black pepper, freshly ground
Directions:

1. Place 20 skewers in a pot of cold water and let them stand for 30 minutes.
2. Mix together the ginger and garlic in a small bowl.
3. Transfer half of the mixture into a large bowl. Add 2 tablespoons of the oil, stir and add the shrimp.
4. Gently stir to evenly coat the shrimp and refrigerate, covered, for at least 30 minutes.

5. Cover the remaining garlic-ginger mixture with cling film and place in the refrigerator.
6. Heat the grill to medium and coat the grates with the oil.
7. Add the plum and green tomatoes to a bowl, add the remaining oil and season with the salt and pepper.
8. Grill the tomatoes, cut side up, until charred and the pulp is tender, about 5- 6 minutes for the plum tomatoes and 10 minutes for the green tomatoes. Remove and let them cool.
9. Remove the skins and seeds from the tomatoes. Thinly chop the pulp and add to the bowl with the reserved garlic-ginger mixture. Stir in the jalapeño, cilantro, basil, lime juice.
10. Season the shrimp with salt and pepper, and thread onto the skewers by piercing through the tail and top. One shrimp per skewer.
11. Grill the shrimp until opaque throughout, about 2-3 minutes each side.
12. Transfer the shrimp skewers onto a platter and serve with a bowl of the relish.

Italian Chicken Soup

This is a very healthy and tasty soup. The addition of mozzarella in this recipe adds more value to this dish. Kids will absolutely adore this soup!

Preparation time: 10 minutes
Cooking time: 60 minutes
Serves: 7

Ingredients:

1 medium onion, chopped
1 garlic clove, minced
4 cups water
1 lb (454g) boneless, skinless chicken breasts, cubed
1 can (800g) Italian tomatoes, crushed
1 can (400g) chicken stock
1 medium green pepper, chopped
1 small carrot, thinly sliced
½ tablespoon red pepper flakes, crushed
1 medium sweet red pepper, chopped
1 celery rib, thinly sliced
3 tablespoons Parmesan cheese, grated
1 teaspoon Italian seasoning
7 tablespoons mozzarella cheese, shredded
¼ tablespoon salt
¼ tablespoon pepper

Directions:

1. Coat a large saucepan with cooking spray.
2. Place the chicken in the pan and cook over a medium heat until pale, 6-7 minutes.
3. Remove the chicken from the pan, transfer to a bowl and cover to keep warm.
4. Add the peppers, carrot, celery and onion to the pan and cook, stirring occasionally, until the vegetables are softened.
5. Add the garlic and cook for a further minute. Pour in the water and add the cooked chicken, tomatoes, chicken stock, Parmesan cheese and seasonings.
6. Once boiling, reduce the heat, remove the lid and simmer for about 40 minutes.
7. Pour the soup into serving bowls, top with the shredded mozzarella and enjoy.

Garlic Parmesan Zucchini and Tomato Bake

This recipe makes a healthy lunch which is easy to assemble as it utilizes ingredients that are always on hand.
Preparation time: 5 minutes
Cooking time: 30 minutes
Serves: 6

Ingredients:
2 large zucchinis, cut into quarters
10oz (280g) grape tomatoes, diced
½ cup Parmesan Cheese, shredded
7 garlic cloves, crushed
1 teaspoon basil, dried
1 teaspoon thyme, dried
1 teaspoon oregano, dried
¾ teaspoon salt
½ teaspoon ground black pepper
⅓ cup parsley or basil, finely chopped
Cooking spray
Directions:

1. Preheat oven to 350°F (175°C) and coat a baking dish with cooking spray.
2. Mix together the cheese, basil, thyme, oregano, cloves, zucchini, tomatoes, salt and pepper in a large bowl.
3. Place the mixture into the prepared baking dish and bake in the oven for 25-30, until the vegetables are tender and the cheese is melted.
4. Remove the bake from the oven, garnish with the chopped basil or parsley, and serve warm.

Greek Salad

This is a refreshing salad recipe ideal for your whole family. This dish features onions, tomatoes, and feta cheese, thus being very healthy and providing you with lots of vitamins.

Preparation time: 5 minutes
Serves: 4
Ingredients:
3 cups tomato, diced
3 teaspoons fresh dill, coarsely chopped
1 teaspoon extra virgin olive oil
1 teaspoon fresh lemon juice
1 teaspoon oregano, dried
¼ cup fresh parsley, coarsely chopped
6 cups Romaine lettuce, shredded
1 cup red onion, thinly sliced
¾ cup feta cheese, crumbled
1 teaspoon capers
1 cucumber, peeled and thinly sliced

Directions:

1. In a small bowl, mix together the olive oil, fresh dill, parsley, lemon juice and oregano.
2. In a large bowl, combine together the lettuce, red onion, capers, feta cheese, cucumber and tomatoes.
3. Pour the prepared dressing over the salad and toss well until coated.
4. Enjoy.

1.

Mediterranean Salmon

Baked salmon topped with healthy vegetables tastes fantastic. Check out this preparation method and see that it is as good as promised.

Preparation time: 5 minutes
Cooking time: 22 minutes
Serves: 4
Ingredients:
4 (6oz/170g) salmon fillets, skinless
2 cups cherry tomatoes, halved
½ cup zucchini, finely chopped
2 tablespoons capers, un-drained
1 tablespoon olive oil
1 (2.25oz/60g) can sliced ripe olives, drained
¼ teaspoon salt
¼ teaspoon black pepper
Cooking spray
Directions;

1. Preheat the oven to 425°F (220° C).
2. Season the fish with the salt and pepper on both sides.
3. Gently oil a baking dish with the cooking spray and arrange the fish fillets on the tray.
4. In a bowl, combine the cherry tomatoes, zucchini, capers and olive oil. Stir to mix well before pouring this mixture over the fish.
5. Bake in the oven for 20-22 minutes, or until the fish is cooked through.

Low Carb Tasty Stuffed Bell Peppers

This is a healthy low carb dish made from green bell peppers, ground beef, tomatoes and cheese, and it is loaded with spices. Saffron and cinnamon give a delicate flavor to this amazing dish.

Preparation time: 20 minutes
Cooking time: 25 minutes
Serves: 6
Ingredients:
4-6 green bell peppers
1 lb extra lean ground beef, or 1 lb ground beef
1 small onion, minced
1 tablespoon olive oil
½ teaspoon salt
¼ teaspoon pepper
2 garlic cloves, minced
½ teaspoon ground cumin
½ teaspoon turmeric
1 teaspoon cinnamon
½ teaspoon saffron
1 medium ripe tomato, chopped
tablespoon fresh lemon juice
4oz (120g) feta cheese, crumbled
2 tablespoons grated parmesan cheese

Directions:

1. Remove the tops from the green bell peppers and gently seed them.
2. Place the peppers in a pot of salted boiling water and let them stand for 5 minutes.
3. Meanwhile, add the olive oil to a large frying pan and set over a medium-high heat.
4. When it begins to shimmer, add the onion and garlic and

sauté for 1 minute.
5. Add the ground beef, cumin, turmeric, saffron, and cinnamon and cook for about 10 minutes, stirring occasionally.
6. Once the meat is almost done stir in the tomato. Let the dish cook until the beef is cooked through. Set aside to cool.
7. Arrange the peppers in a roasting pan. Spoon the beef mixture into the peppers and sprinkle with the parmesan and feta cheese.
8. Cover the roasting pan with foil and bake in the oven at 350°F (170°C) for about 15 minutes.
9. Remove the foil and cook for another 10 minutes.
10. Enjoy.

Spinach Salad with Chicken, Avocado and Goat Cheese

A tasty and healthy salad for those who love classic Mediterranean flavors.

Preparation time: 20 minutes
Cooking time: 0
Serves: 4
Ingredients:
8 cups (1 bag) chopped spinach
1 cup cherry or pear tomatoes, halved
1½ cups cooked chicken, chopped
1 large avocado, sliced
⅓ cup crumbled goat or feta cheese
¼ cup toasted pine nuts
3 tablespoons white wine vinegar
2 tablespoons extra virgin olive oil
1 tablespoon Dijon mustard
salt and freshly ground black pepper, to taste

Directions:

1. Add the chopped spinach to a large salad bowl. Add the cut tomatoes, avocado, chicken, cheese and toasted nuts.
2. In a small bowl, combine together the wine vinegar, olive oil and Dijon Mustard, and season with the salt and pepper.
3. Add the dressing to the salad bowl and mix to combine.
4. Let the salad stand for at least 15 minutes and enjoy.

Spinach Stuffed Chicken Breasts

This is a tasty and healthy recipe that can be served as either a side dish or as a light main dish!

Preparation time: 25 minutes
Cooking time: 60 minutes
Serves: 4
Ingredients:
1 (10oz) package frozen chopped spinach, thawed and drained
½ cup crumbled feta cheese
2 cloves garlic, chopped
4 skinless, boneless chicken breasts
4 slices bacon

- **Directions**:

1. Preheat the oven to 375ºF (190ºC).
2. Mix together the feta cheese, spinach, and garlic in a medium mixing bowl. Set aside.
3. Using a knife, gently open the chicken breasts like a butterfly wing.
4. Put a spoonful of the prepared spinach mixture into each chicken breast.
5. Top with a piece of bacon, wrap and secure with a toothpick.
6. Arrange the folded breasts in a rimmed roasting pan and cover.
7. Bake in the oven for 55-60 minutes, or until the chicken juices run clear.
8. Let the chicken breasts cool for 5-10 minutes and serve warm.

Portobello Mushrooms with Mediterranean Stuffing

I am sure these stuffed mushrooms will quickly become a favorite. Hot, warm or cool, they are always absolutely delicious.

Preparation time: 10 minutes
Cooking time: 35 minutes
Serves: 4
Ingredients:
4 (4-inch) Portobello mushrooms about ¾ lb)
¼ cup onion, finely chopped
¼ cup celery, finely chopped
¼ cup carrot, finely chopped
¼ cup red bell pepper, finely chopped
¼ cup green bell pepper, finely chopped
¼ teaspoon dried Italian seasoning
2 garlic cloves, minced
Cooking spray
½ cup vegetable broth
½ cup (2oz) feta cheese, crumbled
3 tablespoons low-fat balsamic vinaigrette, divided
4 teaspoons grated fresh Parmesan cheese
¼ teaspoon black pepper
4 cups mixed salad greens

Directions:

1. Preheat oven to 350°F (175°C).
2. Remove the stems from the mushrooms and finely cut them to fill ¼ cup. Discard the remaining stems.
3. In a medium bowl, combine ¼ cup of chopped onion, carrot, celery, green bell pepper and red bell pepper.
4. Add the chopped mushroom stems, garlic and Italian seasoning and mix to blend.

5. Coat a large frying pan with cooking spray and set over a medium heat.
6. Add the mixed chopped vegetables and cook for about 10 minutes, or until the vegetables begin to soften.
7. Transfer the mixture into a large bowl.
8. Gradually add the broth and toss to coat.
9. Finally, add the feta and gently mix to combine.
10. Using a spoon, remove the brown gills from the undersides of the mushroom caps, and discard.
11. Gently coat the baking sheet with cooking spray and place the mushroom caps onto it, stem side up. Slightly brush the mushrooms with 1 tablespoon of the vinaigrette.
12. Sprinkle with parmesan cheese and ground black pepper. Top each mushroom cap with ½ cup cooked vegetable mixture.
13. Bake in the oven for 20-25 minutes, or until the mushrooms are softened.
14. Mix together 1 cup of the greens and 2 tablespoons of vinaigrette in a bowl. Place the greens mixture on serving plates and top each serving with one stuffed mushroom.

Roasted Vegetables with Lamb

This tasty dish with roasted vegetables and lamb is nutritious and filling. Just make it and enjoy.

Preparation time: 10 minutes
Cooking time: 30 minutes
Serves: 4
Ingredients:
1 tablespoon olive oil
9oz (250g) lean lamb fillet, trimmed of any fat and thinly sliced
5oz (140g) shallots, halved
2 large zucchinis, cut into chunks
½ teaspoon ground cumin
½ teaspoon paprika
½ teaspoon ground cilantro
1 red, 1 orange and 1 green pepper, cut into chunks
1 garlic clove, sliced
¾ cup vegetable stock
1 cup cherry tomatoes
Handful of cilantro leaves, roughly chopped
Salt and pepper, to taste
Directions:

1. Add the oil to a large griddle and set over a high heat.
2. Add the shallots and lamb and cook for 3-4 minutes until golden in color.
3. Add the zucchinis and cook for about 5 minutes, until just tender.
4. Stir in the cumin, paprika and cilantro.
5. Add the garlic and peppers, reduce the heat to medium and cook for about 5 minutes, until the peppers are tender.
6. Add the tomatoes and vegetable stock and simmer, covered, for 12-15 minutes, stirring frequently.

7. Sprinkle the dish with the roughly chopped cilantro and serve.

Chapter 4
Ketogenic Mediterranean Dinner Recipes
Mediterranean Low-carb "Risotto"

This tasty and healthy recipe can be made in a very short time. Make sure you have all the ingredients on hand and give it a try.

Preparation time: 5 minutes

Cooking time: 23 minutes

Serves: 4

Ingredients:

1 medium head cauliflower (4 cups cauliflower "rice")

4 (1.3 lb/600g) medium chicken breasts, skinless and boneless, cut

¼ cup coconut milk

2 cloves garlic, mashed

½ cup pesto sauce

Zest of ¼ lemon

2 tablespoons basil, oregano and thyme, freshly chopped

2 tablespoons oregano, freshly chopped

2 tablespoons thyme, freshly chopped

2 tablespoons olive oil

Pinch of freshly ground black pepper

½ teaspoon sea salt (or more to taste)

1 cup parmesan cheese, grated

Directions:

1. To make the cauliflower "rice", remove the leaves and core of the cauliflower.
2. Cut into pieces and wash in cold water and drain.
3. Transfer to a blender and pulse until finely ground and it looks like rice.
4. Coat a large skillet with the olive oil and set over a medium-high heat.
5. Add the chicken pieces to the pan and cook for 12-15

minutes, turning 1-2 times, until golden on all sides.
6. Remove from the pan and set aside.
7. Add the olive oil to a large saucepan and place over a medium heat.
8. Add the lemon zest and mashed garlic and sauté for a few seconds, until golden brown.
9. Add the ground cauliflower ("cauli-rice") to the pan and sauté, stirring regularly, for 4-5 minutes, or to the degree of your preferred doneness.
10. Stir in the coconut milk and chopped herbs, and cook for another 2-3 minutes.
11. Season with the freshly ground black pepper and salt.
12. Add the cooked chicken and parmesan cheese, stir, and remove the pan from the heat.
13. Enjoy!

Mediterranean Tilapia with Olive and Almond Tapenade

This dish is guaranteed to become a big winner recipe in your new diet cookbook.

Preparation time: 10 minutes
Cooking time: 10 minutes
Serves: 4
Ingredients:
4 tilapia fillets
2 teaspoons Mediterranean Seasoning
½ teaspoon salt
2 teaspoons olive oil
⅓ cup roasted almonds (whole) or ¼ cup slivered almonds
½ cup olives
1 teaspoon lemon juice
1 teaspoon Mediterranean Seasoning
¼ teaspoon minced garlic
2 tablespoons olive oil
2 tablespoons sun dried tomatoes
Directions:

1. Season the fish with salt and Mediterranean seasoning on one side and lightly press with your fingers.
2. Add 2 teaspoons of olive oil to a large frying pan and set over a moderate heat.
3. Put the fish in the heated pan, seasoned side down, and fry for about 5 minutes, then flip over to brown the other side.
4. Meanwhile, place the almond in a blender and pulse until coarsely ground.
5. Add the lemon juice, garlic, olives, seasoning and oil and pulse for a few seconds.
6. Add the tomato pieces, give a stir and set aside.
7. Once the fish is done, transfer to a serving plate, top each fillet

with the prepared olive mixture and serve.

Salmon with a Warm Tomato-Olive Salad

This recipe has an amazing combination of flavors. As you enjoy your favorite healthy dishes from this book you will realize that The Ketogenic Mediterranean Diet is the best!

Preparation time: 15 min
Cooking time: 10 min
Serves: 4
Ingredients:
5 tablespoons extra virgin olive oil, plus more for brushing
1 tablespoon, plus 1 teaspoon, red wine vinegar
1 tablespoon honey
¼ teaspoon red pepper flakes
Kosher salt
4 (6oz) salmon fillets (about 1¼ inches thick)
1 clove garlic, coarsely chopped
½ cup kalamata olives, pitted and coarsely chopped
2 medium beefsteak tomatoes, cut into 1-inch chunks
1 cup sliced celery (inner stalks with leaves)
¼ cup fresh mint, roughly chopped

Directions

1. Preheat the broiler.
2. In a small bowl, combine together 2 tablespoons of olive oil, the honey, 1 teaspoon vinegar, red pepper flakes and 1 teaspoon salt.
3. Place the salmon, skin-side down, on a baking dish lined with foil.
4. Coat the fish with the honey glaze.
5. Broil until golden brown and the fish flakes easily, for about 5 minutes.
6. Place the garlic on a cutting board, season with a pinch of salt and, using the flat side of a knife, press into a paste.
7. Add the remaining 3 tablespoons of olive oil, garlic paste, olives and 1 tablespoon vinegar to a medium saucepan and set over a medium-high heat.
8. Once it begins to bubble, remove from the heat.
9. Transfer the sauce to a medium salad bowl.
10. Stir in the celery, tomatoes and mint.
11. Flavor with the salt, and stir to coat.
12. Place the salmon onto a serving plate, add the tomato salad and enjoy.

Pork Tenderloin with Olive-Mustard Tapenade

Olives are one of the healthiest ingredients in Mediterranean cooking. They also make this dish outstanding in terms of texture and taste.

Preparation time: 10 minutes
Cooking time: 15 minutes
Serves: 4
Ingredients:
1 (1 lb/454g) pork tenderloin, trimmed and cut
½ teaspoon salt
¼ teaspoon black pepper
¼ teaspoon ground fennel
Cooking spray
¼ cup kalamata olives, chopped and pitted
¼ cup green olives, chopped and pitted
1 tablespoon fresh parsley, chopped
1 tablespoon Dijon mustard
2 teaspoons balsamic vinegar
½ teaspoon bottled garlic, minced
Directions:

1. Place a large frying pan over a medium-high heat.
2. Cut the pork into ½-inch thick round pieces.
3. In a small cup, combine the salt, pepper and fennel, and rub over the pork.
4. Gently drizzle the pork with the cooking spray.
5. Add the seasoned pork to the large frying pan and roast for 5 minutes on each side, until the pork acquires golden crust and it is cooked through.
6. Meanwhile, in a small bowl, mix together the Dijon mustard, balsamic vinegar, green olives, kalamata olives, garlic and parsley.
7. Place the pork onto a serving plate, top with the olive mixture

and enjoy.

Italian Sausage, Peppers and Onions

Sure, this spicy fried Italian sausage with garlic, oregano and basil will become a favorite dish.

Preparation time: 15 minutes
Cooking time: 25 minutes
Serves: 6
Ingredients:

6 (4oz/120g) links sweet Italian sausage
2 tablespoons olive oil
1 yellow onion, sliced
½ red onion, sliced
4 cloves garlic, minced
1 large red bell pepper, sliced
1 green bell pepper, sliced
1 teaspoon dried basil
1 teaspoon dried oregano
¼ cup white wine

- **Directions**

1. Heat a large frying pan over a medium heat.
2. Add the sausage and fry until brown on all sides.
3. Transfer to a cutting board and slice.
4. Add the olive oil to a medium frying pan and set over a medium-high heat.
5. Sauté the red onion, yellow onion and garlic for about 3 minutes.
6. Add the green and red bell peppers, and sprinkle with oregano and basil.
7. Pour in the white wine and cook until the onions and peppers

---

1. http://allrecipes.com/Recipe/Italian-Sausage-Soup/Detail.aspx?nextItemId=76808&position=-1&prop24=RD_RecipeArrow_Left

have softened, stirring frequently, for 5-6 minutes.
8. Return the sausage slices to the pan, reduce the heat and simmer, covered, for about 12 minutes, until the sausage is heated through.

Grilled Pesto Shrimp Skewers

Parmigiano cheese, garlic and basil leaves provide a great tasting variation on these crispy shrimp skewers.

Preparation time: 2 hours 10 minutes (including marinating time)
Cooking time: 10 minutes
Serves: 7
Ingredients:
1 cup fresh basil leaves, chopped
1 clove garlic
¼ cup grated Parmigiano Reggiano
3 tablespoons olive oil
1½ lbs jumbo shrimp, peeled and deveined (weight after peeled)
Kosher salt, to taste
Freshly ground pepper, to taste
7 wooden skewers

Directions:

1. Place the wooden skewers in water and let them stand for about 30 minutes.
2. Place the garlic, basil, Parmigiano cheese, salt and pepper in a blender and pulse until finely ground. When pulsing, pour in the olive oil in a slow steady steam.
3. In a medium bowl, place together the pesto and raw shrimp and let them stand for 1-2 hours.
4. Combine the raw shrimp with the pesto and marinate a few hours in a bowl.
5. Place the shrimp onto the skewers.
6. Prepare an outdoor grill, or set an indoor grill pan under a medium-low heat.
7. Gently coat the grates with the oil.
8. Arrange the skewers on the grill and cook for 4 minutes per side.
9. Once the shrimp is cooked through, remove from the heat and let them stand for a few minutes to cool.
10. Enjoy.

Grilled Chicken with Tomato Mixture

This is a very hearty and spicy meal made with chicken and mozzarella cheese. My family loves this so I always double the recipe!

Preparation time: 5 minutes
Cooking time: 10 minutes
Serves: 4
Ingredients:
4 boneless, skinless chicken breasts
Pinch of salt
¼ cup balsamic vinegar
¼ cup extra virgin olive oil
8 slices fresh mozzarella cheese
4 Roma tomatoes, seeded and diced
8 fresh basil leaves, stacked and cut
3 cloves fresh garlic, minced
1 tablespoon balsamic vinegar

Directions:

1. Coat a grill pan with cooking spray and set under a medium heat.
2. In a bowl, mix together the ¼ cup olive oil and ¼ cup balsamic vinegar.
3. Season the chicken breasts with the salt, and coat with the balsamic mixture. Place the chicken on the heated grill pan.
4. Grill for about 5 minutes before turning to brown the other side.
5. Coat with the additional balsamic mixture, if needed, and grill for another 5 minutes.
6. 3 minutes prior to full readiness, top each chicken piece with 2 slices of cheese.
7. Place the tomatoes, 1 tablespoon balsamic vinegar, salt and

garlic in a medium bowl and mix to combine.
8. Place the warm grilled chicken on a serving dish and spoon the tomato mixture over the chicken.
9. Enjoy.

Zucchini, Tomato and Mozzarella Pie

I often make this tasty dish and my family always crave for more. The zucchini combines nicely with the tomatoes and mozzarella cheese.

Preparation time: 25 minutes
Cooking time: 40 minutes
Serves: 4
Ingredients:
3 medium zucchinis
Sea salt, as needed
4-5 cloves garlic, minced
Freshly ground pepper, to taste
Extra virgin olive oil
8oz mozzarella, sliced
3 medium vine-ripe or heirloom tomatoes, sliced
Freshly chopped basil, to taste
Directions:

1. Preheat the oven to 375°F (180°C).
2. Halve the zucchini and thinly cut lengthwise into strips
3. Season with salt and pepper and let them sit in a colander for 9-10 minutes.
4. Transfer to paper towels to drain.
5. In an even layer, arrange the zucchini in a baking dish and sprinkle with the minced garlic and pepper.
6. Sprinkle with olive oil and top with the mozzarella slices, followed by the tomato slices.
7. Sprinkle with the chopped basil, sea salt and pepper.
8. Bake the mixture in the oven until the zucchini has softened, for about 40 minutes.
9. Remove from the oven and let it sit for 10 minutes
10. Slice into squares and enjoy.

Baked Cod with Roasted Vegetables

Fish likes spice! Garlic, black pepper and citrus juice make this dish an unforgettable experience, which is, by the way, not difficult to achieve.

Preparation time: 20 minutes
Cooking time: 45 minutes
Serves: 2
Ingredients:
Half a head of purple cabbage, sliced thinly
1 sweet or red onion, sliced
4 cloves garlic, chopped
1½ cups broccoli florets
1 green sweet pepper, sliced into strips
2 carrots, sliced into strips
⅓ cup extra virgin olive oil
¼ cup balsamic vinegar
⅓ cup apricot preserves
2 cloves garlic, minced
Sea salt, to taste
Freshly ground pepper, to taste
½ teaspoon mild or hot curry
A dab of honey mustard (optional)
For the fish:
2 single cod fillets (or one large fillet, cut in half)
Extra virgin olive oil
2-3 cloves garlic, chopped
A squeeze of citrus (lemon, lime or orange)
Sea salt, to taste
Freshly ground pepper, to taste

Directions:

1. Preheat the oven to 400°F (200°C) and position the rack on the middle of the oven.
2. In a large bowl, place together the sliced cabbage, onion, chopped garlic, broccoli, carrots and pepper.
3. In a separate small bowl, combine the olive oil, vinegar, apricot preserves, minced garlic, curry, salt, pepper and honey (if using).
4. Pour the mixture over the vegetables and toss to coat.
5. Place the vegetables in the roasting pan and transfer to the oven.
6. Let the vegetables roast in the preheated oven until crisp-tender, for about 45 minutes.
7. When the vegetables are nearly done, or 10 minutes prior to full readiness, start cooking the fish.
8. Put the fillets in a baking dish, top with the garlic, and drizzle with the citrus juice and olive oil. Season with the salt and pepper.
9. Set the rack in the upper position in the oven.
10. Bake the fish until opaque throughout, for about 8-10 minutes.
11. Place the fish on a serving plate alongside the roasted vegetables. Pour any remaining roasting sauce over the top of the fish and vegetables, and serve.

Mediterranean Chicken and Vegetable Kebabs

This is a must-try for poultry lovers. Make sure the chicken breasts are well marinated, which will add an unforgettable taste to the whole dish.

Preparation time: 40 minutes
Cooking time: 10 minutes
Serves: 6
Ingredients:
¼ cup fresh lemon juice
2 tablespoons freshly chopped Oregano, or 2 teaspoons dried oregano
2 tablespoons olive oil
1½ pounds skinless, boneless chicken breast, cut into 24 strips
18 (½-inch-thick) slices zucchini
1 fennel bulb, cut into 12 wedges
12 garlic cloves, peeled
½ teaspoon salt
¼ teaspoon black pepper
Cooking spray

Directions:

1. Place the chicken, fennel bulb, zucchini, olive oil, lemon juice and oregano into a zip-top, heavy duty plastic bag. Seal the bag and shake well to coat.
2. Place in the refrigerator and let it marinate for 25 minutes.
3. Remove the chicken from the plastic bag and discard the marinade.
4. Prepare the grill.
5. Add the garlic cloves to a pot of boiling water and cook for 3 minutes.
6. Remove the garlic from the water and cool.
7. Thread 3 zucchini slices, 4 chicken strips, 2 garlic cloves and 2 fennel wedges, alternately, onto the skewers and season with salt and pepper.
8. Gently coat the grill grate with cooking spray and arrange the skewers on it.
9. Grill the kebabs for about 10 minutes, until golden-brown, turning 1-2 times.

Seared Mediterranean Tuna Steaks

This is a wonderful fish dish, full of authentic Mediterranean flavors. It is prepared in a short time, yet gives you an unforgettable experience.

Preparation time: 5 minutes
Cooking time: 10 minutes
Serves: 4
Ingredients:
4 (6oz/180g) tuna steaks (about ¾ inch thick)
½ teaspoon salt
½ teaspoon ground cilantro
⅛ teaspoon black pepper
Cooking spray
1½ cups seeded tomato, chopped
¼ cup green onions, chopped
3 tablespoons fresh parsley, chopped
1 tablespoon capers, drained
1 tablespoon extra virgin olive oil
1 tablespoon lemon juice
½ teaspoon bottled minced garlic
12 kalamata olives, pitted and chopped
Directions:

1. Coat a large frying pan with cooking spray and set over a medium-high heat.
2. Season the tuna steaks with cilantro, ¼ teaspoon salt and pepper.
3. Place the fish in the heated pan and fry for about 5 minutes per side, until golden brown.
4. Meanwhile, in a small bowl, mix together the tomato, onions, capers, kalamata olives, garlic, lemon juice, olive oil and fresh parsley.

5. Place the cooked fish on a serving plate, top with the tomato mixture and enjoy.

Beef Tenderloin with Mustard and Herbs

Every time I prepare this simple dish for my guests I am always asked for the recipe!

Preparation time: 15 minutes
Cooking time: 25 minutes
Serves: 10

- **Ingredients**:

1 (2½ lb) beef tenderloin, trimmed
Cooking spray
1 teaspoon salt
1 teaspoon freshly ground black pepper
⅓ cup fresh parsley, finely chopped
2 tablespoons fresh thyme, chopped
1½ tablespoons fresh rosemary, finely chopped
3 tablespoons Dijon mustard

Directions:

1. Preheat the grill on a high heat.
2. Gently sprinkle the beef with cooking spray and season with salt and pepper.
3. Oil the grill grate with cooking spray and place the beef on the grate.
4. Reduce the heat to medium and grill the beef for about 25 minutes, until the beef acquires a golden brown crust on all sides.
5. Let the beef cool for 5- 10 minutes.
6. In an even layer, spread the chopped thyme, parsley, and rosemary in a flat platter. Coat the grilled beef with Dijon mustard and place into the platter with the herbs.
7. Gently roll the beef over the herbs until it is evenly coated.
8. Slice the beef and enjoy.

Chapter 5
Ketogenic Mediterranean Snack Recipes
Low Carb Cabbage Patties

These cabbage patties will melt in your mouth. Make sure you have all the ingredients at hand and get ready for this special experience.

Preparation time: 5 minutes
Cooking time: 10 minutes
Serves: 2
Ingredients:
2 cups cabbage, thinly sliced
1 egg
1 green onion, chopped
1 tablespoon olive oil
Salt and pepper, to taste
Directions:

1. In a medium bowl, mix together the cabbage, onion and egg, and season with salt and pepper.
2. Add the oil to a large frying pan and set over a medium-high heat.
3. Using your hands, shape two patties from the cabbage mixture and fry in the heated pan, for about 4-5 minutes.
4. Flip over to brown the other side, then serve.

Low Carb Turkey Patties

Almost everyone loves turkey, and this method of preparation, with dried sage leaves and ginger, will not leave anyone disappointed.

Preparation time: 5 minutes
Cooking time: 25 minutes
Serves: 4-6

- **Ingredients**:

2 lbs (908g) lean ground turkey
1½ teaspoons salt
1 teaspoon dried sage leaves
1 teaspoon pepper
½ teaspoon ground ginger
½ teaspoon cayenne pepper

- **Directions**:

1. Place the ground turkey in a large bowl, add the cayenne pepper, ginger, salt, pepper and sage, and mix well to combine.
2. Heat a non-stick skillet over a medium-high heat.
3. Shape 16 round patties and fry in the skillet for about 5 minutes per side, until golden brown on all sides.

Zucchini Parmesan Crisps

These crispy zucchini slices are a great treat for any gathering. The process is very easy and the taste is unforgettable.

Preparation time: 10 minutes
Cooking time: 25 minutes
Serves: 4
Ingredients:

1 lb (454g) zucchini or squash (about 2 medium-sized)

¼ cup shredded parmesan

1 tablespoon olive oil

¼ teaspoon kosher salt

Freshly ground pepper, to taste

Directions:

1. Preheat the oven to 400°F (200°C).
2. Line two baking dishes with parchment paper and gently coat with the cooking spray.
3. Thinly slice the zucchini into rounds.
4. Drizzle the rounds with the oil.
5. In a shallow bowl, mix together the parmesan, salt and pepper.
6. Coat both sides of the zucchini rounds with the parmesan mixture.
7. Arrange the coated rounds in a single layer on the prepared baking dishes.
8. Bake in the oven for about 25 minutes, until golden brown.

Tuna and Zucchini Patties

This is an easy and tasty way to serve fish. Your guests will really appreciate it!

Preparation time: 5 minutes
Cooking time: 15 minutes
Serves: 6
Ingredients:
1 (3oz/115g) can of tuna in olive oil
1 large zucchini, grated
2 large eggs
20g (0.7oz) coconut flour
2 teaspoons dried chili flakes, or 1 whole fresh chili, finely chopped and fried
½ teaspoon salt
½ teaspoon black or red pepper
⅛ teaspoon xanthan gum
Olive oil (for frying)

Directions:

1. Using a fork, crumble the tuna in a medium bowl.
2. Add the eggs and zucchini and stir well to combine.
3. In a small cup, mix together the coconut flour, salt and pepper, xantham gum and chili flakes.
4. Combine the coconut flour with the spices and other dry ingredients, and add to the tuna mixture.
5. Combine the zucchini mixture with the coconut flour mixture and stir well until blended.
6. Let the mixture sit for 5 minutes.
7. Add the olive oil to a large skillet and set over a medium heat.
8. Once sizzling, spoon the mixture into the skillet to make 6 large round patties.
9. Let the patties cook for about 6 minutes, then turn to brown

the other side. Transfer the patties to paper towels to drain.
10. Arrange the patties on a serving dish and enjoy.

Roasted Broccoli and Tomatoes

This is a quick and tasty way to serve the broccoli. This dish can be served as a snack or as a great side dish to any meal.

Preparation time: 5 minutes
Cooking time: 12 minutes
Serves: 4
Ingredients:
12oz (350g) broccoli crowns, trimmed and cut into bite-size florets (about 4 cups)
1 cup grape tomatoes
2 tablespoons extra virgin olive oil
2 cloves garlic, minced
¼ teaspoon salt
½ teaspoon lemon zest
1 tablespoon lemon juice
10 pitted black olives, sliced
1 teaspoon dried oregano
2 teaspoons capers, rinsed (optional)
Directions:

1. Preheat oven to 450°F (220°C).
2. In a large bowl, combine the tomatoes, broccoli, garlic and salt.
3. Add the olive oil and mix to combine.
4. Transfer the tomato mixture to a baking dish, spread evenly and bake for 10-12 minutes, until crisp-tender and brown.
5. In a large mixing bowl, mix the oregano, olives, lemon zest, juice and capers (if using).
6. Add the roasted vegetables and toss to coat.
7. Serve warm and enjoy.

Mediterranean Canapés with Cranberries and Goat Cheese

This is a perfect treat if you are a defender of healthy food and lifestyle, so keep this recipe safe!

Preparation time: 10 minutes
Cooking time: 5 minutes
Serves: 8
Ingredients:
1 teaspoon olive oil
24 walnut halves
⅛ teaspoon ground cinnamon
8oz (230g) fresh goat cheese
24 thin rounds of cucumber
½ cup cranberries, dried
1 teaspoon fresh thyme, chopped
Coarse salt
Ground pepper
Directions:

1. Preheat oven to 375ºF (190ºC).
2. Place the walnuts on a baking tray, drizzle with 1 teaspoon oil, and sprinkle with salt, pepper and cinnamon.
3. Bake in the oven until light brown and fragrant, for about 5 minutes. Remove from the oven and let it cool.
4. Arrange the cucumber slices on a serving plate and season with salt and pepper.
5. In a medium bowl, combine the cheese and 2 tablespoons of water.
6. Toss in the cranberries, stir, and then add the thyme, salt and pepper.
7. Spread the goat cheese mixture onto the cucumber slices, garnish with walnuts and enjoy.

Tomato-Basil Skewers

A great refreshing summer snack that is quick and very easy to prepare.

Preparation time: 10 minutes
Cooking time: 0 minutes
Makes: 16 pieces

Ingredients:
16 small, fresh mozzarella balls
16 fresh basil leaves
16 cherry tomatoes
Extra-virgin olive oil, to drizzle
Coarse salt & freshly ground pepper, to taste

Directions:

1. Place the tomatoes, mozzarella and basil on small wooden skewers.
2. Season with salt and pepper, and drizzle with a little olive oil.
3. Arrange the skewers onto a plate and serve.

Conclusion

Thanks for downloading this book!

hope this book has provided you with comprehensive and valuable advice that you can use to improve your health and weight. We also hope that this book will help you to change your perception for the word "diet", making it sound less severe and more enticing.

hope this cookbook was able to help you to prepare more delicious and healthier meals with The Ketogenic Mediterranean Diet recipes.

Thank you and good luck!

www.ingramcontent.com/pod-product-compliance
Lightning Source LLC
LaVergne TN
LVHW041935070526
838199LV00051BA/2794